MEDICAL PROCEDURES, TESTING AND TECHNOLOGY

NEW DEVELOPMENTS IN KNEE PROSTHESIS RESEARCH

MEDICAL PROCEDURES, TESTING AND TECHNOLOGY

Additional books in this series can be found on Nova's website under the Series tab.

Additional e-books in this series can be found on Nova's website under the e-book tab.

MEDICAL PROCEDURES, TESTING AND TECHNOLOGY

NEW DEVELOPMENTS IN KNEE PROSTHESIS RESEARCH

JANICE STEWART
EDITOR

NOVA BIOMEDICAL

New York

Library of Congress Cataloging-in-Publication Data

ISBN: 978-1-63482-700-3
Library of Congress Control Number: 2015937681

Published by Nova Science Publishers, Inc. † New York

Contents

Preface

In this book, the complete development of an external intelligent knee prosthesis created by the Mechatronics Research Group (MRG) was presented. This project brought out several advances in the prosthetic field which the authors discuss in detail. The second chapter examines the use of finite element modeling for understanding knee prosthesis biomechanics, fundamental to answering clinical question in the field. Also looked at are the basic characteristics of knee prostheses that must be complied with in order to provide a safe and biomechanical performance to its users during walking. Other chapters present the main results from a project whose main focus was to evaluate the tibial inserts wear and to obtain the possibility to control the total knee prosthesis (TKPs) wear process; whether screening and decolonization (S&D) is effective in reducing the rate of postoperative infection after elective knee joint arthroplasty and whether it's cost-effective; and finally, a review of the current literature, as well as some personal experiences, on assessing the reliability of patient specific instrument system in total knee arthroplasty (TKA).

Chapter 1 – In this chapter, the complete development of an external intelligent knee prosthesis created by the Mechatronics Research Group (MRG) of the Simón Bolívar University is presented. This project has brought out several advances in the prosthetic field, especially referring external intelligent knee prostheses, such as bio-inspired shape of the chassis, characterization of gait cycle from accelerometer data captured on the legs during walking, continuous control strategies borrowed from nature and robotics, and more recently, a variable impedance actuator, which allows the MRG prosthesis to go far beyond the starting expectations. All these were novel features regarding the state-of-the-art by the time they were introduced, but of course, all this did not happen at a time; on the contrary, the project has experienced an evolution from the first passive prototype equipped with a commercial magneto-rheological (MR) actuator, to the most recent active one, equipped with a variable stiffness actuator created by us. This chapter explains most of the details of such evolution process, going through the motivations of the project, the technical developments that have emerged along the way, and the flaws and limitations of the approaches tested and how these have been overcome. Somehow this work is a compilation of a series of articles published by the co-authors on this matter, but on the other hand, it is a completely new text never published before, as this presents all the content that has emerged from this project up-to-now as a whole for the first time.

Chapter 2 – According to a survey done in the literature on the field until 2010, design of 4-bar mechanisms for polycentric knee prostheses was performed heuristically. Therefore, the main motivation of this work was to determine aspects of the design process on this kind of prosthetic devices suitable of a technical approach, which could go far beyond from a simple empirical point of view. Knee prostheses must comply several basic characteristics in order to provide a safe and biomechanical performance to its user during walking, these are: 1. stability during load response, 2. easy flexion during late stance and pre-swing, 3. recover of extension during late swing before next contact, and 4. proper resistance to critical loading. From these, 1 and 2 might be related to the location of the instantaneous center of rotation (ICR) of the prosthesis with regard to the ground reaction force (GRF) line during the stance phase of gait cycle. The third aspect requires the proper analysis of forces and moments of the assistant extension mechanism (AEM) respect to the ICR and the latter requires a detailed structural stress analysis of the device. For proper kinematical functioning, dimensions of the 4 linkages of the mechanism must be set, as well as the angular position of the prosthesis on the leg. This renders a multi-dimensional search problem that is complex to solve. Nonetheless, artificial intelligence techniques have emerged as a very good alternative to carry out this kind of searches. In particular, genetic algorithms (GAs) perform a search with bias in a multi-dimensional space of solutions. In this work, the aforementioned dimensions of the mechanism, targeting a specific trajectory of the ICR, were gauged by a particularly programmed GA integrated with gait analysis data on a computing platform. Later, a structural analysis of the prosthesis was performed via finite element method, according to the requirements of the standard ISO 10328. And finally, a functional prototype was manufactured and adapted to two unilateral transfemoral amputees, which allowed assessing the performance of the design qualitatively, using questionnaire, and quantitatively, via gait analysis. This work is based on a series of articles published by the co-authors on this matter, but at the same time, it is a new text never published before as a whole, as this presents all the content brought out by this project up-to-now for the first time.

Chapter 3 – The total knee prosthesis (TKP) must allow complex movements in a cyclic charge regime: flexion-extension (FE), antero-posterior translation (APT) and internal-external rotation (IER). Still, its major drawback is failure of a tibial insert due to the subsurface cracking and delamination wear. This chapter presents the main results of a project whose main focus was to evaluate the tibial inserts wear and to obtain the possibility to control the TKPs wear process. First, some retrieved TKPs were analysed revealing the loss of functionality, because the polyethylene tibial insert was dislocated. Next, theoretical wear studies were performed on tibial tray, based on FEM modelling, and practical studies on ball/flat couple. By applying FE and APT movements under constant compressive loading, the results showed that the fracture of tibial tray was preponderantly caused by the adhesive wear and material fatigue. A thorough analysis was conducted with focus on phenomenon evolution, from adhesive wear pitting followed by delamination and even breaking of the insert. The failure mechanism proved being a combination of the high level of loading during normal activities and a non-conforming contact between the femoral condyles and tibial insert. The question that arises is: Could be this phenomenon evaluated quantitatively a priori?

In order to determine the occurrence of wear in high risk areas, a predictive method was used by combining the Finite Element Analyses of contact mechanism and transfer of load in articulation, with a summation technique based on damage score estimation. Finite element simulations were performed to dynamically determine the contact area, and the contact pressure resulting in normal walking, stairs ascending and stairs descending. The finite element model used a modern contact mechanism, including friction between the metallic femoral condyles and the tibial polyethylene insert. Summation was adopted in order to consider the cumulative effect of all activities, based on their frequency and the magnitude of the determined damage function. The computed surface of cumulative maximum damage that traverse the layers of the polyethylene insert could be identified as the cracking surface. The conclusion was that a partial answer to the question stated before could be achieved by the presented method, which was able to determine the path of the subsequent failure of the polyethylene inserts.

Based on these results, it was established the basis for implementing control strategies for a Knee Prosthesis Simulator (KPS), by Programmable Logical Controllers in Open Architecture structure. This complex procedure allowed transferring real loads from the patient artificial knee to the KPS control system, through kinematic acquisition, evaluation of joint loadings and dynamic simulation of joint contact. Practically, the data resulting from motion analysis of the patient activities would be processed by a specialized code which would determine the motion dynamic loadings of the joint. Based on data, a detailed joint tribological model would allow contact dynamics determination and generate the customized evolution of each of the controlled KPS degrees of freedoms. The use of this method would improve the accuracy of lifetime predictions, based on the experimental data obtained in a KPS.

Chapter 4 – Biomechanical numerical models in orthopedic research are currently becoming more and more frequent, complex and comprehensive. In this context, finite element analysis of biomechanical models has consistently increased in the last decades. The growing trend in the use of such numerical technique is indeed strongly correlated with the increasing and the easiest access to computational resources and, parallel to this, with the development of more sophisticated data handling algorithms. In fact, looking to the past, the use of finite element analysis in the field of biomechanics was mainly limited to simplistic approaches, such as bi-dimensional models, considering mainly linear analyses, and investigation of single structures or tissue types only. Nowadays, fully three-dimensional, nonlinear, multi-structures and tissues, and even multi-joint systems, can be also easily implemented in the simulation. More specifically, for a knee with an implant (e.g., total knee arthroplasty (TKA), unicondilar knee arthroplasty (UKA) or patello-femoral joint), the model aims to replicate the behavior of three-dimensional biological structures, like bones, cartilage and ligaments, coupled with non-biological knee components made of different synthetic materials. An additional complexity in knee modeling is provided by the huge variability inherent to the field. This variability is due to the vast range of different kinematics and contact forces that could be induced by the variety of prosthesis designs, in different patients, and under specific motor tasks. Due to the multiplicity of these aspects, the use of finite element modeling is of foremost importance; in fact, it allows to obtain qualitative guesses and qualitative data that cannot be provided by any other method (such as in-vitro experimental tests or gait analysis) such as the stresses distribution for bone and prosthesis components under different conditions, and contact forces interactions, both for generic and patient-specific solutions. These outputs, coupled with clinical outputs, allow to relate, for example, stress changes, from the physiological to a knee with a prosthesis and to a bone mineral density changes in the patients, allowing to formulate possible answers to common unsolved clinical questions. An added value derived by the use of finite element analysis is the possibility to characterize performances of prosthesis designs in restoring knee functions and maintaining long-term mechanical integrity for different patients and in agreement with different surgeon requests. In more general terms, the use of finite element modeling in the understanding of knee prosthesis biomechanics is fundamental to answer clinical questions, to improve and predict clinical outputs, to provide more surgeon-friendly guidelines and, last but not least, to improve TKA success and avoid critical situations. This modeling procedure can help bridging the gap between surgeons and engineers, aiming in the improving of the biomechanical research on knee prosthesis.

Chapter 5 – *Purpose:* In recent years, patient-specific instruments (PSI) has been introduced with the aim to reduce the overall costs of the implants, minimising the size and number of instruments required, and also reducing surgery time. The purpose of this study was to perform a review of the current literature, as well as to report about our personal experience, to assess reliability of patient specific instrument system in total knee arthroplasty (TKA). *Method:* A literature review was conducted of PSI system reviewing articles related to coronal alignment, clinical knee and function scores, cost, patient satisfaction and complications. Results: Studies have reported incidences of coronal alignment $\geq 3°$ from neutral in TKAs performed with patient-specific cutting guides ranging from 6 % to 31 %. *Conclusion:* PSI seem not to be able to result in the same degree of accuracy as for the CAS system, while comparing well with standard manual technique with respect to component positioning and overall lower axis, in particular in the sagittal plane. In cases in which custom-made cutting jigs were used, we recommend performing an accurate control of the alignment before and after any cuts and in any further step of the procedure, in order to avoid possible outliers.

Chapter 6 – *Background:* Although some have advocated screening (nasal swab using polymerase chain reaction (PCR)-based testing), followed by decolonization using a 5 to 14-days course of nasal mucopirocin (2 per cent nasal ointment) for methicillin resistant *Staphylococcus aureus* (MRSA), it is unclear whether screening and decolonization (S&D) among knee joint arthroplasty patients reduce surgical site infections (SSIs) *Purpose:* The purpose of this chapter is to review the literature with the aim of answering the following three questions: 1) Is S&D effective in reducing the rate of postoperative infection after elective knee joint arthroplasty? 2) Is S&D cost-effective? 3) What is the durability of decolonization? *Methods*: The search engines were MedLine (PubMed), Google Scholar and the Cochrane Library. The keywords used were: preoperative MRSA screening. 8008 papers were found until 25 October 2014 (7910 in Google Scholar, 97 in MedLine and one in the Cochrane Library). Of those, only eighteen were selected and reviewed because they were strictly focused on the question of this article. *Results:* The types of studies reported have a low level of evidence (level III, level IV). Most of them are prospective case series (level IV), although some of them are systematic reviews of level III studies. Regarding the efficacy of decolonization, the literature shows a tendency toward fewer MRSA infections after elective knee joint arthroplasty. Decolonization has shown to be strongly cost-effective. Regarding the durability of decolonization, in a study 33% of postoperative arthroplasty patients tested positive for SA colonization at 3 to 30 months after surgery. *Conclusions:* The review of the literature found a tendency toward fewer MRSA infections after knee joint arthroplasty when S&D was used. Decolonization is strongly cost-effective procedure. Regarding the durability of decolonization, 33% of patients tested positive for MRSA 3 to 30 months after surgery. However, most of these studies were underpowered. Larger, randomized, controlled studies are needed to confirm the apparent efficacy of decolonization.

In: New Developments in Knee Prosthesis Research
Editor: Janice Stewart
ISBN: 978-1-63482-700-3

Chapter 1

Evolution of External Intelligent Knee Prosthesis: From Passive to Active Through Variable Compliance Actuation

Rafael R. Torrealba[1,2], Samuel B. Udelman[1,2], José Cappelletto[1], Leonardo Fermín[1], Gerardo Fernández-López[1], Juan C. Grieco[1], Lilibeth A. Zambrano[2], Gabriel Messingher[2] and Eliane Andara[2]

Mechatronics[1] and Biomechanics[2] Research Groups,
Simón Bolívar University, Caracas, Venezuela

Abstract

In this chapter, the complete development of an external intelligent knee prosthesis created by the Mechatronics Research Group (MRG) of the Simón Bolívar University is presented. This project has brought out several advances in the prosthetic field, especially referring external intelligent knee prostheses, such as bio-inspired shape of the chassis, characterization of gait cycle from accelerometer data captured on the legs during walking, continuous control strategies borrowed from nature and robotics, and more recently, a variable impedance actuator, which allows the MRG prosthesis to go far beyond the starting expectations. All these were novel features regarding the state-of-the-art by the time they were introduced, but of course, all this did not happen at a time; on the contrary, the project has experienced an evolution from the first passive prototype equipped with a commercial magneto-rheological (MR) actuator, to the most recent active one, equipped with a variable stiffness actuator created by us. This chapter explains most of the details of such evolution process, going through the motivations of the project, the technical developments that have emerged along the way, and the flaws and limitations of the approaches tested and how these have been overcome. Somehow this work is a compilation of a series of articles published by the co-authors on this matter, but on the other hand, it is a completely new text never published before, as this presents all the content that has emerged from this project up-to-now as a whole for the first time.

1. Introduction

In 2007, the MRG of the Simón Bolívar University started a project to develop an intelligent prosthetic knee for transfemoral amputees. The idea was to launch a new research line specifically tailored to the development of ortho-prosthetic devices and technology (DODT). Both upper and lower limbs were considered to start with, but it was found that the latters had a higher incidence in terms of population affected with amputations, not only in Venezuela but also in the rest of the world [1,2]. Then, once situated on lower limbs, the next question that emerged was what joint to work with: hip, knee or ankle. In particular, from biomechanics of human gait, it is seen that hip and ankle are the motors that move the body forward during walking, while knee plays a fundamental role in terms of flow of energy between joints as well as enabling the natural kinematics of biped locomotion [3]. Therefore, hip or ankle prostheses would need an active system to motorize the joint, while a knee prosthesis could offer a good performance basically equipped with a passive system that dissipates energy in a conveniently-controlled way along gait cycle.

Furthermore, the incidence of patients that need a hip prosthesis is really low when compared to cases in which a prosthetic knee or ankle is required. Regarding the ankle joint, current prosthetic feet that store energy during load response and then deliver it to push-off the leg into pre-swing, seem to offer quite an acceptable performance in order to assist the dynamics of gait. Most of these feet present a solid ankle, so there is no articulated connection at the joint and therefore, designing an ankle prosthesis was deemed desirable but not compulsory. Hence, the knee was selected as the joint to work with, to develop a prosthesis to help amputees to recover their possibility of walking.

On the other hand, mechanical and intelligent knee prostheses already existed and were available at the market by that moment, but taking advantage of the knowledge and capabilities of the MRG regarding mechatronics and design, it was decided to carry out the development of an intelligent knee prosthesis instead of a merely mechanical one. The term 'intelligent' in lower-limb prostheses indicates the prosthesis is able to change its response during walking. This concept arose once electronics was applied to the prosthetic field by Prof. Flowers and his collaborators at the MIT, during the 1970s [4-6]. Subsequently, there has been a series of technical developments all aimed at creating a knee prosthesis capable of mimicking the natural kinetics of a human leg. A complete review of the latters was performed in 2008 and is summarized in the following section of this chapter [7].

2. Review of Research on Knee Prostheses

To start this project, the first step was setting a detailed state-of-the-art of scientific research towards the development of knee prostheses. By doing this, authors came up with a complete reference frame that allowed them to have a clear comprehension of the research done up to then [7]. A remarkable feature of this review was the identification of three scientific research lines regarding the development of knee prostheses, each one dealing with: the design of knee prostheses; the performance assessment of these prostheses; and the creation of control strategies for these prostheses which use electronics to control their performance. Given the complexity of reproducing a natural gait on a prosthetic device, regardless it is a function that brain controls practically unconsciously, scientific research has approached such problem from different sides.

2.1. Design of Knee Prostheses

This first research line outlined a close relationship between scientific research and commercial launching of prostheses since the end of World War I [8,9], until the 1990s, when the first versions of intelligent prosthetic knees came into the market [10-12]. There was shown a complete evolution initiating with the constant-friction and friction-brake designs back in the 1920s, passing by the fluid-controlled prostheses introduced by Hans Mauch in the 1950s [13-15], until the application of electronics to control these devices from the 1970s [4-6]. The first knees presented serious problems to the possibility of walking at different speeds, and/or on uneven surfaces. Later, with the introduction of fluid in actuators, high-resistive torques for giving the user the security and stability required during the stance phase were possible. And also, due to the intrinsic property of fluidness of the liquid contained in the actuator, it resulted that knee flexions during the swing, and returns to the extended position before heel strike in a more harmonious way for a wider range of cadences. Finally, with the intelligent knee prostheses, the major adaptability of their technology began to be exploited, especially to help above-knee amputees to walk again.

2.2. Performance Assessment of Knee Prostheses

On the second research line, it was aimed at quantifying how good a given prosthesis is. In this sense, a gait lab takes particular importance being an especially tailored facility to acquire and process data related to human walking. Consequently, curves of movements of different joints are generated and thus reconstruction of gait cycle is possible [16,17]. Regarding lower limbs, it is usual to measure angular positions of the joints, as well as reaction forces from the ground. Then, making use of dynamic models, it is possible to determine also torques and powers applied on each joint. In prostheses assessment, results obtained when walking with the prosthesis are compared with results obtained from a sound leg in terms of these variables, and thus, it is set how far the prosthetic performance is from the natural one, in a very accurate way [18-20]. Similarly, assessing a prosthesis performance is done by comparison with others. Indeed, it is commonly used since most of publications which evaluate performance of a prosthesis does it [21-24].

Another application of gait labs is capturing and processing electromyographic (EMG) signals, i.e., electrical signals coming from muscles. This is achieved through electrodes placed on points of interest, and it is of special relevance given the great potential these signals have for doing an eventual control on a prosthetic device [25]. Likewise, comparisons are made considering also variables of energy. It means that metabolic consumption using different prostheses is measured at gait lab, and from these values, conclusions are obtained regarding the reachable efficiency with each design [26-28]. Finally, there were also publications which took patient opinion for setting conclusions instead of using gait analysis. These might be less scientific, but being the patient the user of the assessed device, these are not less valid at all [29,30].

2.3. Control Strategies of Intelligent Knee Prostheses

As last, regarding the third research line, it basically explained the finite-state control, a.k.a. soft control, which was the only strategy applied by commercial prostheses by the time the review was carried out. Classical control, based on a dynamic-mathematical model of the locomotive system, has been claimed to result extremely complex, less robust and hence, very difficult to implement on real-time [31]. On the contrary, 'soft control' is a non-analytical strategy based on a group of pre-stated rules that, combined with information about certain controlling parameters related to natural and prosthetic gait, allows to take control actions on the prosthesis actuator. We will go deeper into this matter in the next sections, but let's say in advance that this implies that the prosthetic device is equipped with sensors to try to identify the instant of gait cycle in which the user is. Then, once an instant is identified, it is associated with a state, which once again is attached to a pre-stated rule that turns into a determined control action.

Nonetheless, other approaches had been also proposed. For instance, use of central pattern generators (CPGs) was introduced to develop an algorithm that reproduces biped-locomotion [32], different machine learning techniques for automatic generation of control rules on locomotion had been also implemented [33], and even a search of intrinsic angular momentum primitives of human gait had been carried out [34]. Regarding EMG signals, it was known that information carried by these might be useful for identifying user intention and hence, controlling a prosthesis. Several works had addressed this matter [35-37], especially in upper limbs. On lower limbs, however, there was no commercial prosthesis which used an EMG-based control strategy yet. According to [25], there were several difficulties in practical implementation of this kind of technology, especially for identifying and capturing EMG signals of interest, processing these signals, and characterizing the adaptation of muscular activity according to the prosthetic device used by the patient. Not to mention the muscular fatigue effects, which can cause additional problems in the control of myoelectric prostheses [38]. Nowadays, nevertheless, scientific research continues making efforts in applying EMG-based control strategies on lower limb prostheses as it is the natural way of putting the user's volition in command of the prosthesis performance [39-41].

The review ended introducing cybernetic prostheses, which will be not only a physical substitution for a loss limb, but also, will be controlled by the same function used by natural limb through the human nervous system, without being connected to it. Robotic systems have been working with concepts such as CPGs, for generating joint trajectories and synchronizing them, to reproduce the different gait modes biologically possible in walking robots [42-44]. These CPGs have been found in nature, as biological neural networks which control locomotion in vertebrate and invertebrate animals [45], and recently, robotics has been using virtual CPGs to control locomotion in walking robots [46], including humanoid ones [47]. Cybernetic prostheses will take advantage of this knowledge too, and will apply such bio-inspired concepts, for example to generate the joint trajectory of a knee prosthesis in all possible walking modes, allowing to control its performance in a much more smooth and reliable way.

To close this section, Figure 1 presents a bar-plot indicating the three aforementioned research lines identified in this review, besides a further division of them showing the number of references found for each in percentage.

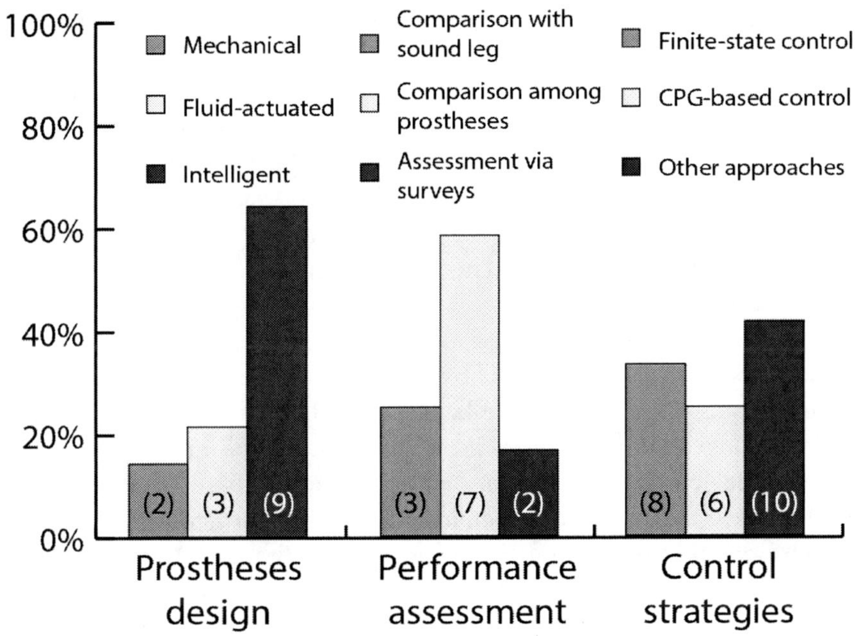

Figure 1. Research lines identified in the state-of-the-art review. Based on Torrealba R. R., Fernández-López G. & Grieco J. C. (2008): Towards the development of knee prostheses: review of current researches. Kybernetes: The International Journal of Systems & Cybernetics, Vol. 37, No. 9/10, pp. 1561-1576.

3. Mechanical Design Introducing a Bio-Inspired Shape

Being an intelligent prosthesis a mechatronic device, its design has to take into account both mechanical and electronic parts. Moreover, to put the horses before the carriage, the mechanical structure should be designed first but always bearing in mind what electronics will be in the final prototype. This in order to go through a smooth design process, instead of a back and forth, never-ending one. The mechanical structure of the prosthesis refers basically to the chassis, which allocates the knee joint mechanism and holds the complete prosthesis as a whole. This physical component is of paramount importance as it is the one that actually substitutes the leg. The prosthesis must assure certain requirements of strength to guarantee the integrity of itself and hence, of the user during walking. As a matter of fact, there is a particular international standard to comply with [48].

3.1. Bio-Inspired Shape Embedded on the Prosthesis

Regarding the shape and finishing of the prosthesis, it is typically used a foam cover over it, once adapted to its user by an orthoprosthetist. This extra cover looks for a more natural aspect of the prosthesis to make it seem a sound human leg. In this project, however, contrary to this common practice, a bio-inspired shape is included directly on the chassis, thus eliminating the need of such extra cosmetic cover. Actually, the use or request of this cover depends on several variables. For instance, it is observed that in more conservative societies people prefer to wrap their prostheses with human-like covers, while on the contrary, in more open-minded societies they like, or at least do not care, to simply expose their prostheses as the biomechatronic devices they are. Likewise, many times it is also found that young users would rather to wear their prostheses without covers, but the older ones prefer the contrary.

3.2. Mechanism and Actuator of the Prosthesis

As to the mechanisms of knee prostheses, there are monocentric and polycentric designs [49]. In the formers, there is a fixed axis over which the flexo-extension of the mechanism occurs, hence it works as a hinge. In the latters, there is an instantaneous center of rotation whose location changes with the flexo-extension angle of the mechanism. Natural human knee presents a polycentric design, but in the present work, however, a monocentric mechanism was preferred in order to simplify the design. Furthermore, it was deemed that electronic control would take care of the adaptations on the prosthesis response in order to make it more human-like. On the other hand, there are passive and active prostheses as well. The first ones only dissipates energy at the joint, while the second ones are also capable of introducing it. Hence, the actuator in the passive prostheses may be a hydraulic or pneumatic cylinder controlled by opening or closing its valves through servomotors, as in the Genium® of Otto Bock [50], or a magneto-rheological brake whose response is modulated by the current intensity that flows through the electromagnetic circuit associated, as happens with the Rheo Knee® of Össur [51]. For the active ones, counting just with the Power Knee® [52] and the Vanderbilt Leg® [53] up-to-now, it is all about electrical motors.

In addition to the monocentric design, the prosthesis here developed was initially passive, equipped with a commercial magneto-rheological (MR) actuator. These actuators offer resistance to motion, and being the torque applied on the knee joint during walking mostly resistive, it made sense to use this kind of actuator for this particular application [19]. The prosthesis was designed in ProENGINEER® Wildfire 3.0. The mechanism consists of three main parts: the chassis, the knee joint and the actuator, as seen in Figure 2. The chassis was designed according to dimensions of the first author's leg; measurements were made by cross-sectioning the leg virtually along the tibia, and then taken into the software to generate the external surface of the chassis.

The interior of the chassis was defined basically to contain the actuator and the knee joint, since the electronics was supposed to be placed outside the prosthesis in this first prototype.

Figure 3 shows a longitudinal cross-section showing the main parts of the mechanism, as well as the axes that connect them, in three different knee angular positions: 0, 45 and 85°.

The prosthesis was designed to use standard commercial adaptors to be coupled with the socket and foot-ankle unit that complete the (transfemoral) lower-limb prosthesis.

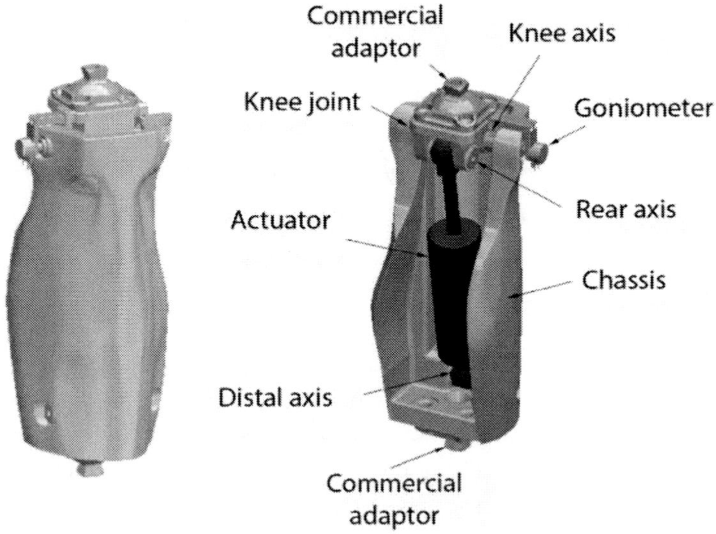

Figure 2. External intelligent knee prosthesis with bio-inspired shape.

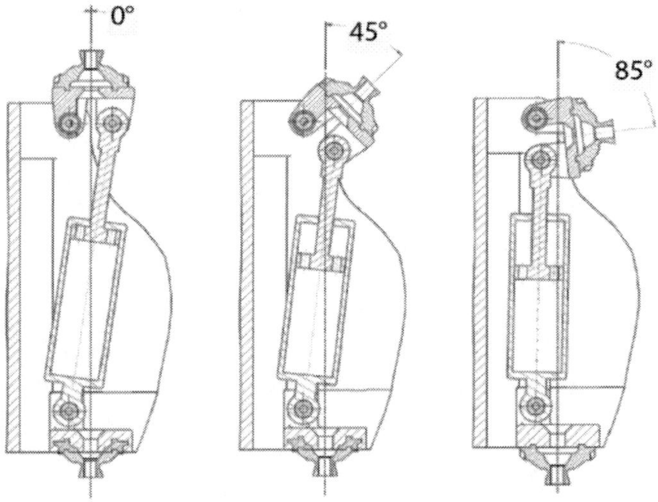

Figure 3. Cross-section of the monocentric mechanism equipped with MR actuator.

3.3. Manufacture of the Prosthesis

The chassis was manufactured with prosthetics and orthotics materials and technology found in a local specialized workshop. The chassis resulted a multilayer material composed of two layers of co-polymer (a mix of polyethylene and polypropylene typically used to laminate prostheses and orthoses), which defined its interior and exterior surfaces, filled with a layer of medium-density polyurethane between both.

Finally, the chassis was laminated with fiberglass in resin to seal the exterior and provide further strength through a very thin but rigid layer. The metallic pieces were manufactured with conventional metal-working machines found locally. The overall weight of the prosthesis was 2,059 g, which was slightly heavier than similar commercial devices, which range between 1,400 and 1,700 g approximately.

4. Accelerometry-Based Human Gait Characterization

As aforementioned, intelligent prostheses execute some sort of control on their response. For that, as any other controller, their microprocessor requires to acquire some inputs to determine the current situation of the prosthesis in order to send a corresponding control action to its actuator. In terms of a lower limb joint, this means that the microprocessor onboard the prosthesis needs to characterize the human gait cycle in order to apply a particular control action. Natural walking consists of a series of successive motions imprinted by muscular contractions on skeleton segments harmoniously orchestrated by the nervous system. Part of this, however, is missing in amputees, and here it is where an intelligent prosthesis must take over and set an actuator response in accordance to the user's intention.

4.1. Innovating Instrumentation of Intelligent Knee Prostheses

By 2007, characterization of gait cycle on intelligent knee prostheses was roughly based on strain gauges located on particular points on the lower limb prosthetic device and a goniometer to measure the knee angle [11,12]. This arrangement allowed to separate stance phase from swing phase and also, differentiate load response from pre-swing along the former, but not much more. Thus, we came out with the idea of using accelerometers [54,55], instead of strain gauges, for characterizing the gait cycle on our prosthesis. It was not the first time that accelerations had been mentioned in studies related to above-knee (A/K) prostheses [28,31], but it did was the first time that acceleration data was used expressly to characterize human gait cycle.

We speculated that being inertial movements of the lower limb segments involved throughout the gait cycle, accelerometer signals should be of special utility to detect gait events, even during swing phase, through which strain gauges, by the way, do not measure anything (as the foot is out of contact with the floor). We were right, and by developing a complete approach to accelerometry-based characterization of gait cycle, we pioneered this field of prosthetic technology [56-58]. Few years later, commercial intelligent prostheses introduced these sensors and current ones are usually equipped with these plus gyroscopes, which are sensors of the same family (inertial sensors) that measure angular velocity of rigid bodies [50,51,59].

4.2. Accelerometry-Based Gait Events Detection

A system was developed for capturing gait data. It consisted of three subsystems, i.e., the sensors and hardware designed for holding these on the leg during walking, the data-acquisition module which was composed of the data-acquisition board and the microcontroller, and a user interface, which allowed us to set some parameters of interest and display results while capturing and saving data. The captured signals were the knee angle and the accelerations at the knee and ankle joints in the sagittal plane. For capturing the knee angle we conditioned an articulated-knee support with a 10 KΩ potentiometer. The accelerations were captured using two bi-axial accelerometers placed at the knee and ankle joints, specifically at the femoral condyles and malleollus height, respectively. We started working with a normal person with two sound legs. Nevertheless, during the trials the instrumentation was placed just on one leg, so the knee support with the potentiometer was placed medially while the accelerometers were placed laterally. In particular, the accelerometers were placed in such a way that the 'y'-axis went along the tibia and the 'x'-axis went perpendicular to it. All the signals were captured at a frequency of 50 Hz and saved as data files for post-processing using MATLAB®. All the algorithms used were developed for obtaining specific results in order to demonstrate if it was possible to identify the different phases of gait cycle, as well as their sub-divisions, using only knee angle and accelerometers data.

Figure 4 shows part of the captured accelerometer data walking on level terrain at self-selected speed. Furthermore, as we did not know the acceleration curve behavior along the gait cycle in advance, while the knee angle behavior was quite known, we also plotted the latter in order to have a reference, which allowed us to relate them to each other. From Figure 4, we made the hypothesis that the heel contact and hence the gait cycle initiates at the negative peak of 'x' acceleration that follows its highest positive one. Also we stated that the toe-off occurs at the second major negative peak of 'x' acceleration, just before this acceleration begins to increase. Then, just working with accelerations and jerks at the ankle joint, plus knee angular position, we were able to obtain every heel contact event and, with it, to identify each gait cycle. The results are shown in Figure 5.

Further analysis was conducted to identify the other six events that occur along the gait cycle. For doing this, in general we worked with ten signals, five directly captured, plus their five derivatives. Theoretically, each of these events initiates a new sub-phase along the gait cycle and in fact, these so-stated sub-phases fit the characterization of gait cycle by Nordin and Frankel [60] in number, although not exactly in percentages stated for each one. According to [60], the gait cycle is divided into seven sub-phases, four for stance phase and three for swing phase. The stance phase is divided into loading response (0–10% of gait cycle), midstance (10–30% of gait cycle), terminal stance (30–50% of gait cycle) and pre-swing (50–60% of gait cycle). The swing phase is divided into initial swing (60–73% of gait cycle), midswing (73–87% of gait cycle) and terminal swing (87–100% of gait cycle).

Leaving aside the heel contact event, which starts the gait cycle, the other six events we identified occurred on average at 8, 40, 52, 61, 70 and 93% of the gait cycle, which led again to four sub-phases in stance and three sub-phases in swing.

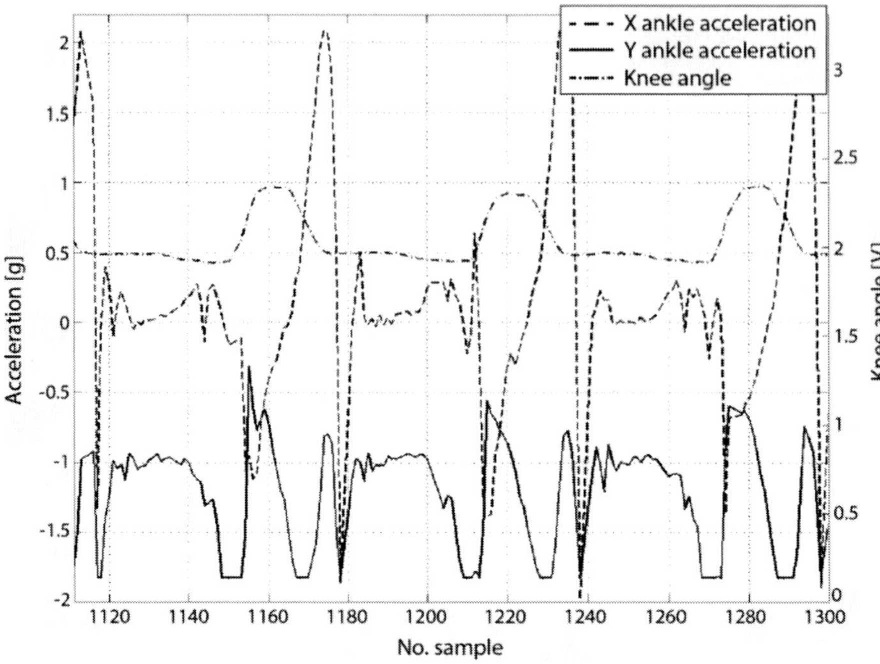

Figure 4. Captured data at ankle joint. Adapted from Torrealba R. R., Castellano J. M., Fernández-López G. & Grieco J. C. (2007): Characterisation of gait cycle from accelerometer data. Electronics Letter, Vol. 43, No. 20, pp. 1066-1068.

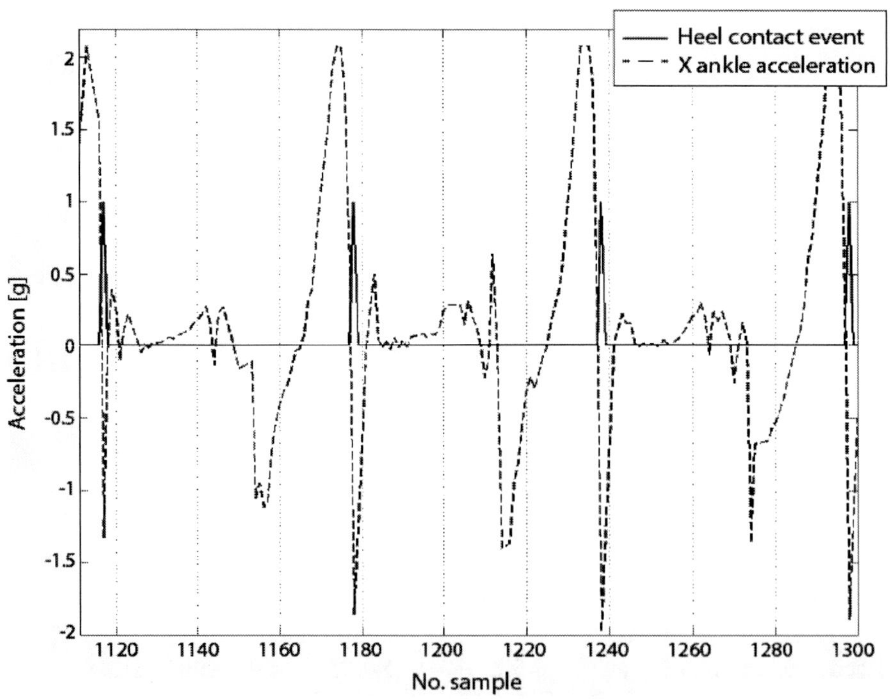

Figure 5. Heel contact identification from 'x' ankle acceleration. Adapted from Torrealba R. R., Castellano J. M., Fernández-López G. & Grieco J. C. (2007): Characterisation of gait cycle from accelerometer data. Electronics Letter, Vol. 43, No. 20, pp. 1066-1068.

The stance sub-phases went from 0 to 8% of gait cycle, from 8 to 40% of gait cycle, from 40 to 52% of gait cycle and from 52 to 61% of gait cycle. Likewise, the swing sub-phases went from 61 to 70% of gait cycle, from 70 to 93% of gait cycle and from 93 to 100% of gait cycle. These events are shown in Figure 6.

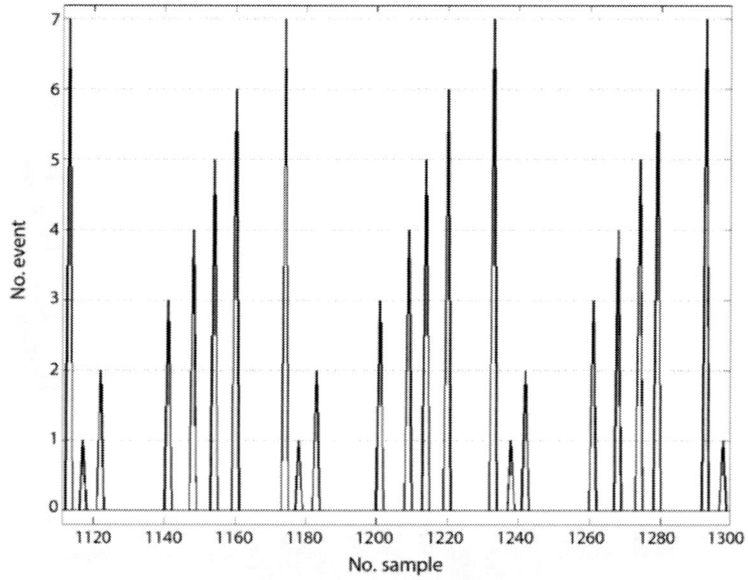

Figure 6. Identified events from acceleration signals. Adapted from Torrealba R. R., Castellano J. M., Fernández-López G. & Grieco J. C. (2007): Characterisation of gait cycle from accelerometer data. Electronics Letter, Vol. 43, No. 20, pp. 1066-1068.

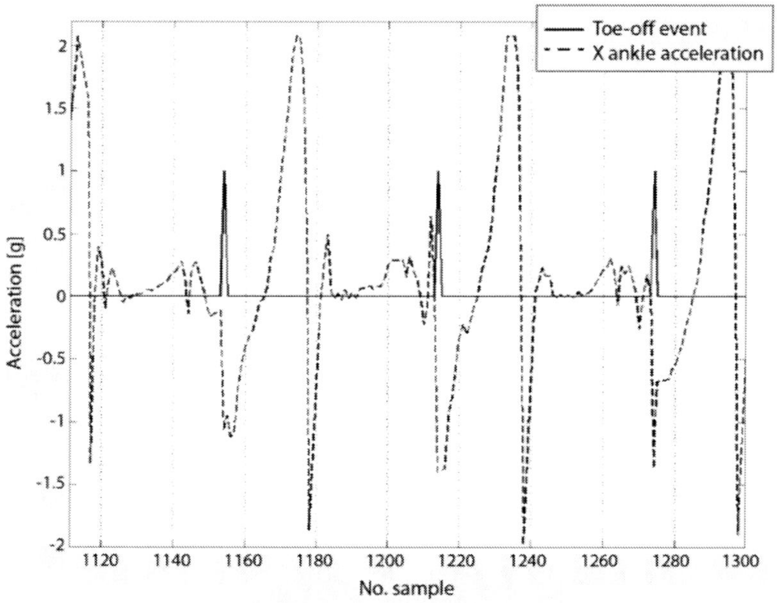

Figure 7. Toe-off identification from 'x' ankle acceleration. Adapted from Torrealba R. R., Castellano J. M., Fernández-López G. & Grieco J. C. (2007): Characterisation of gait cycle from accelerometer data. Electronics Letter, Vol. 43, No. 20, pp. 1066-1068.

Finally from that first work, as seen from the heel-contact-occurrence assumed hypothesis, there resulted an event at 61% of gait cycle, which obviously corresponded to toe-off given that it perfectly matched the standard percentage for this event in human gait. Moreover, this event coincided with the second major negative peak of 'x' acceleration at the ankle joint as initially proposed above for toe-off. This is shown in Figure 7.

4.3. Correlation-Based Gait Cycle Tracker

By then, the accelerometry-based gait events detection algorithm (AGEDA) was based on hand-tuned thresholds. Also, this had been proved only with a healthy person walking at a self-selected speed and automation of the thresholds setting was still required. In addition, the system needed testing with different patients and at variable gait speeds. One of the alternatives studied to overcome the abovementioned situation was a correlation-based gait cycle tracker. A waveform corresponding to a single gait cycle may be extracted as shown in Figure 8a. Using this waveform as a template, it is possible to identify the gait cycle phase. By running the correlation between the template and the actual acceleration signal, an overall surface is obtained as shown in Figure 8b. In this figure, the local minimum along the template axis represents the instant at which the template completely overlaps with the actual signal, therefore indicating the current phase of the gait cycle. In other words, the correlation result allows tracking the progress of the gait cycle continuously, until reaching the next one. As seen, this approach proved good results on data captured from the healthy person walking at constant speed, however, at the end, this technique had to be abandoned because it showed serious limitations dealing with differences between the actual signal and the template, as those coming from gait speed changes, for instance.

4.4. Statistics-Based Gait Events Detection

Once the prosthesis was built, similar waveforms of the accelerometers signals were obtained when testing it with an amputee patient. A solution to automatically adapt the thresholds initially set by hand-tuning emerged through the use of statistics. The original AGEDA was modified to work directly with the signals captured by the accelerometers on the prosthesis, applying their recent statistics to set the corresponding thresholds automatically. The block diagram of the new statistics-based gait event detection algorithm (SGEDA) is shown in Figure 9. The signal conditioning block (SCB) filters out high frequency electrical noise and its outputs enters into the threshold levels setting block (TLSB) and the signal spikes isolation block (SSIB). The TLSB sets the threshold levels based on recent statistics of the corresponding signal. Then, the SSIB applies the corresponding thresholds to every signal in order to isolate the overshot spikes from which gait events are detected. Finally, the local minima (on valleys) or maxima (on peaks) of the signals are determined via differentiation, which are directly the events detected by the algorithm as output of the local minima/maxima calculation block (LMMCB).

The keynote of the SGEDA is the TLSB applied to the accelerometer signals; this is based on the Kaplan-Meier cumulative distribution function (CDF) as implemented by MATLAB®. The histogram and CDF of the accelerometer signals computed from 1,000 samples are plotted in Figure 10. As can be observed, the CDF is very steep for all the signals (see Figs. 10d–f), indicating that most of the data is close to the distribution mean (see Figs. 10a–c). The values located far from the mean correspond to CDF values near 0 or 1, which refer to valleys and peaks, respectively. The CDF of a signal represents the probability that a random variable X is lower than or equal to a value A (set by a percentile) in the sample space. Then, by setting convenient fixed percentiles, it was possible to adjust the level of the thresholds to isolate the peak and valley zones automatically.

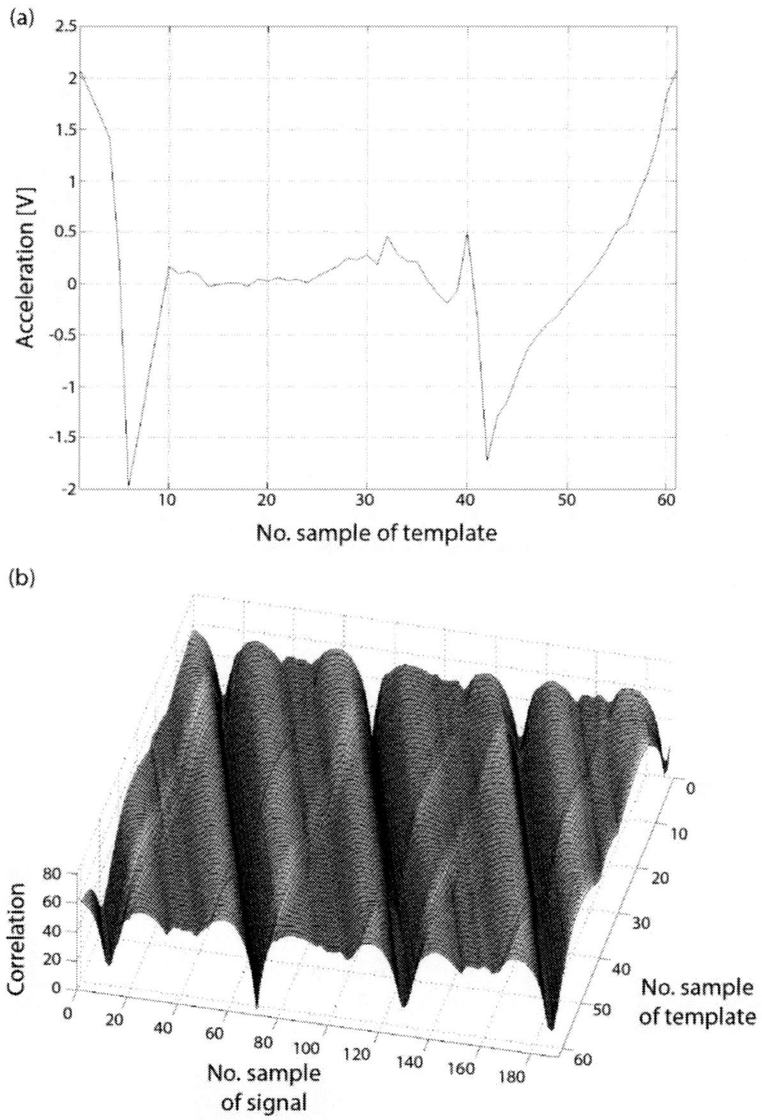

Figure 8. Correlation-based gait cycle tracker: (a) Gait cycle waveform, (b) Correaltion surface. Adapted from Torrealba R. R., Pérez-D'Arpino C., Cappelletto J., Fermín-León L., Fernández-López G. & Grieco J. C. (2010): Through the development of a biomechatronic knee prosthesis for transfemoral amputees: mechanical design and manufacture, human gait characterization, intelligent control strategies and tests. Proceedings of the IEEE International Conference on Robotics and Automation ICRA'2010, Anchorage, AK-USA, pp. 2934-2939.

The acceleration signals used by the SGEDA as conditioned by the SCB are shown in Figure 11. These were captured with the patient walking at 2 kph and the thresholds (percentiles) and events detected in real-time are also shown. In Figure 11b, two different valleys are detected for each gait cycle. The less deep valley corresponds to heel strike (0% of gait cycle) and the deepest one to toe-off (~60% of gait cycle), the two most important events along the gait cycle which determine the start of stance and swing phases, respectively [56].

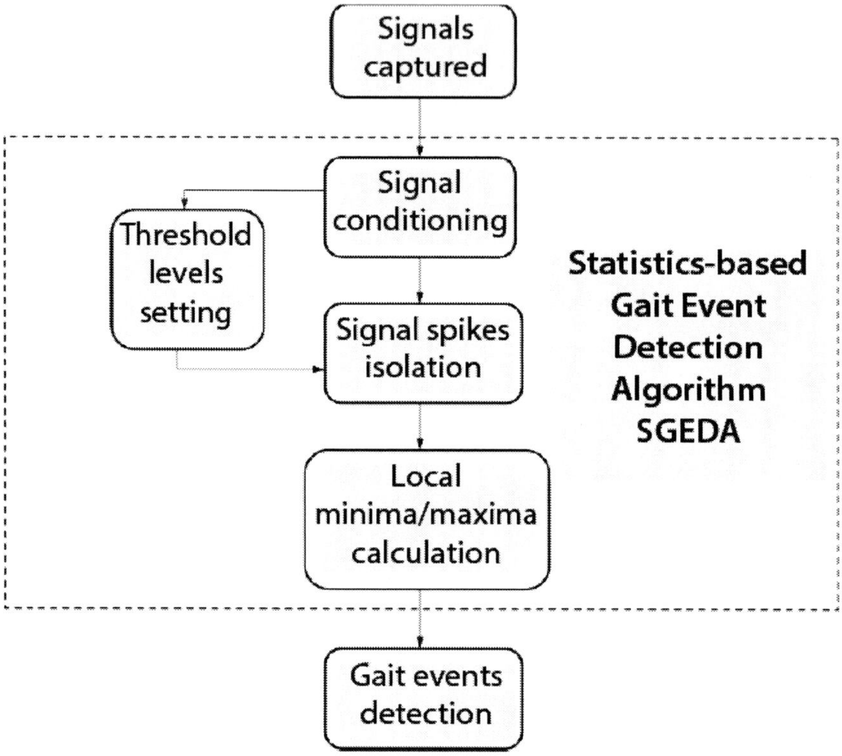

Figure 9. Block diagram of the SGEDA. Adapted from Torrealba R. R., Pérez-D'Arpino C., Cappelletto J., Fermín-León L., Fernández-López G. & Grieco J. C. (2010): Through the development of a biomechatronic knee prosthesis for transfemoral amputees: mechanical design and manufacture, human gait characterization, intelligent control strategies and tests. Proceedings of the IEEE International Conference on Robotics and Automation ICRA'2010, Anchorage, AK-USA, pp. 2934-2939.

For a finite state control, these results would enable one to define different states in terms of percentages of gait cycle. Nevertheless, the final control strategy sought by us would use the events detected for gait frequency and phase estimation only. It must be noticed that the mean of the signals shown in Figure 11 differ from each other but, in order to isolate the peaks and valleys and later detect these as gait events, percentiles are set absolutely regardless of the mean values. This was one of the major assets of the statistics-based technique developed then.

To test the method, two thresholds were applied on the 'x' ankle acceleration while the amplitude of the signal was artificially varied. The thresholds were set at percentiles 7 and 93 to detect the deepest valley and highest peak of the signal only (see Figure 12).

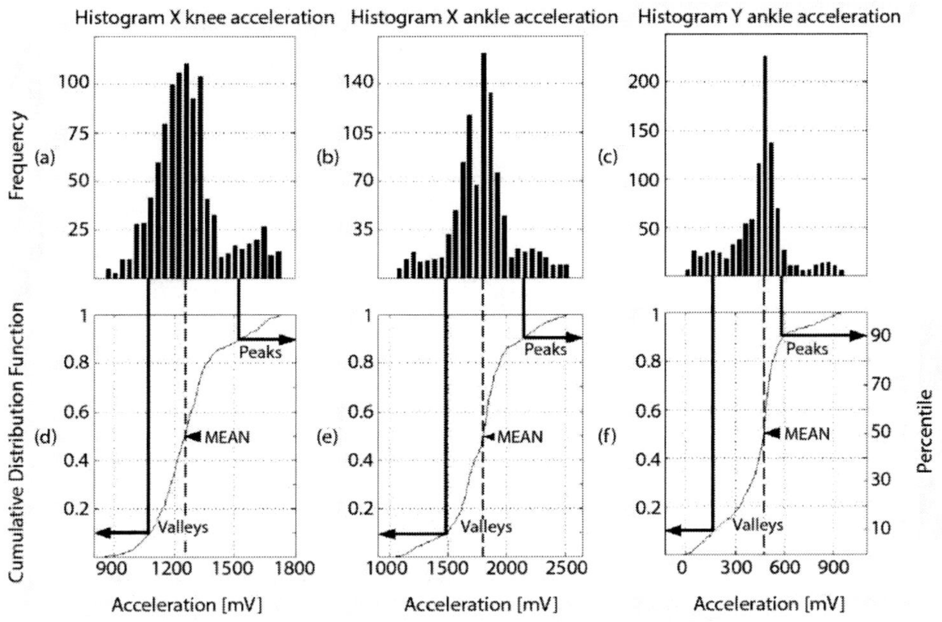

Figure 10. Histogram and cumulative distribution function of accelerometer signals. Adapted from Torrealba R. R., Cappelletto J., Fermín L., Grieco J. C. & Fernández-López G. (2010): Statistics-based technique for automated detection of gait events from accelerometer signals. Electronics Letters, Vol. 46, No. 22, pp. 1483-1485.

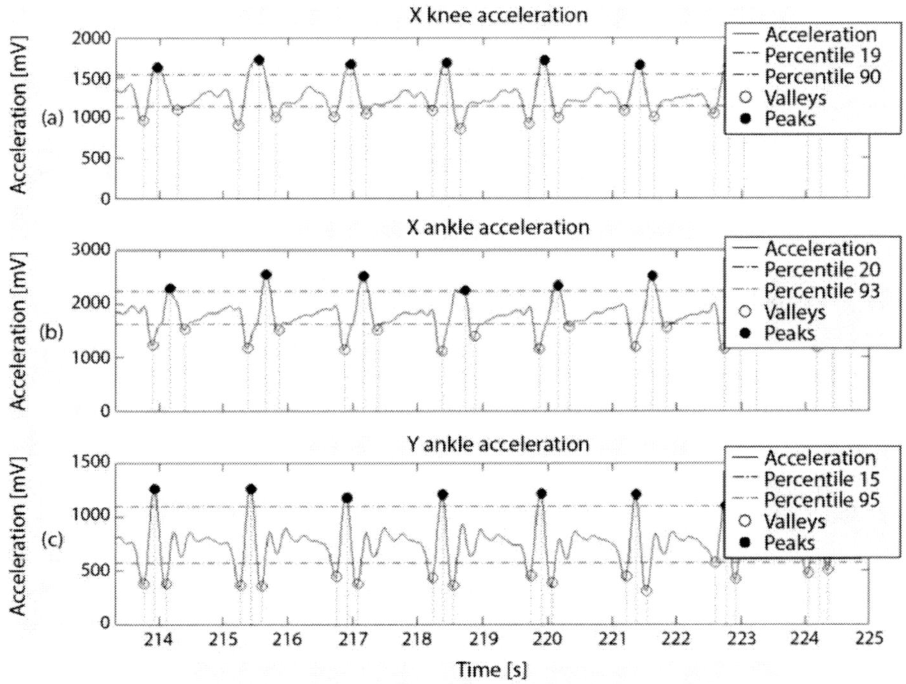

Figure 11. Signals, thresholds and events detected by the SGEDA. Adapted from Torrealba R. R., Cappelletto J., Fermín L., Grieco J. C. & Fernández-López G. (2010): Statistics-based technique for automated detection of gait events from accelerometer signals. Electronics Letters, Vol. 46, No. 22, pp. 1483-1485.

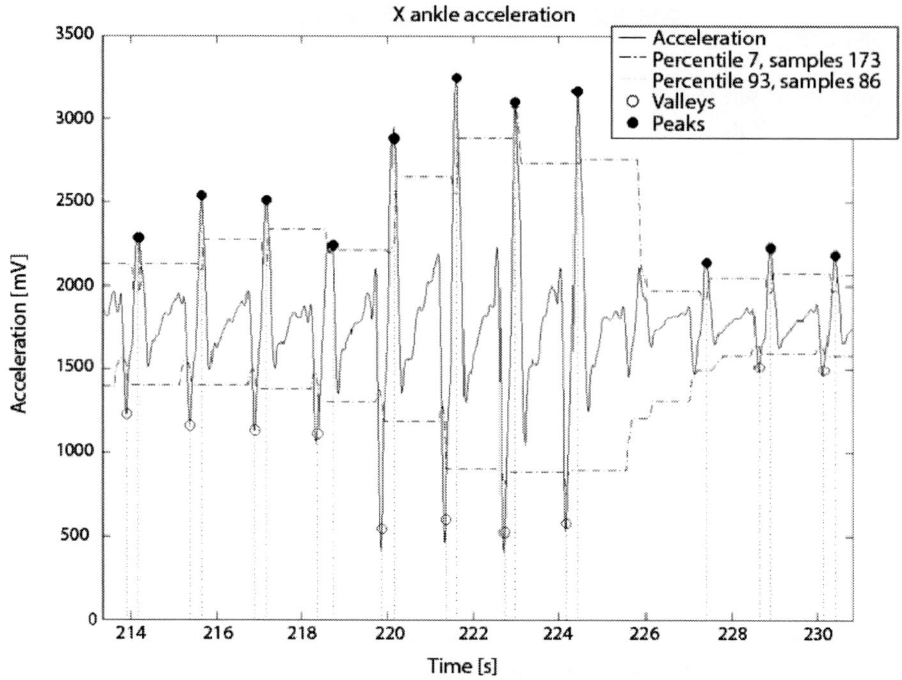

Figure 12. Adaptive response of the SGEDA to amplitude modulation. Adapted from Torrealba R. R., Cappelletto J., Fermín L., Grieco J. C. & Fernández-López G. (2010): Statistics-based technique for automated detection of gait events from accelerometer signals. Electronics Letters, Vol. 46, No. 22, pp. 1483-1485.

The lower threshold was computed from 173 samples whereas the higher one was from 86, to evaluate the sample window size effect. No event was missed when the signal amplitude was doubled, but some were overlooked when it was reduced by half.

As expected, the higher threshold responded faster than the lower one; this means that the lower the number of samples to determine the percentiles to set the thresholds, the faster the adaptive response of the SGEDA was and vice versa. These results made evident the other major asset of this technique, which was its capability to handle scale factors.

Finally, frequency modulation is shown in Figure 13 while the same previous two thresholds were applied on the 'x' ankle acceleration signal. It is observed that the deepest valley was always detected from the lower threshold regardless of the frequency modulation. However, the higher threshold failed to detect only the highest peak of the signal when it was modulated at half the sampling frequency (30 Hz).

In this case, the threshold was adapted so fast that the second higher peak began to be detected as well, as seen from 219 to 229 s. From the signal modulated at twice the sampling frequency (120 Hz), it is observed that the higher threshold detected only the highest peak of the signal again. In other words, a threshold applied according to a percentile set from a given number of samples at a certain frequency, will work for higher frequencies also but not necessarily for lower ones.

Conclusions of that work claimed that the two major assets of the technique presented were the automated setting of the thresholds used to isolate the spikes, regardless of the signal offset, and the easy-adaptive response of the thresholds to scale factors. The sensitivity of the algorithm depended on the number of samples taken into account to calculate the percentiles used to set the threshold levels. In general, the algorithm performance was accurate, but however, for safety reasons additional filtering might be included, to avoid any false or missing detection when controlling a lower limb prosthesis.

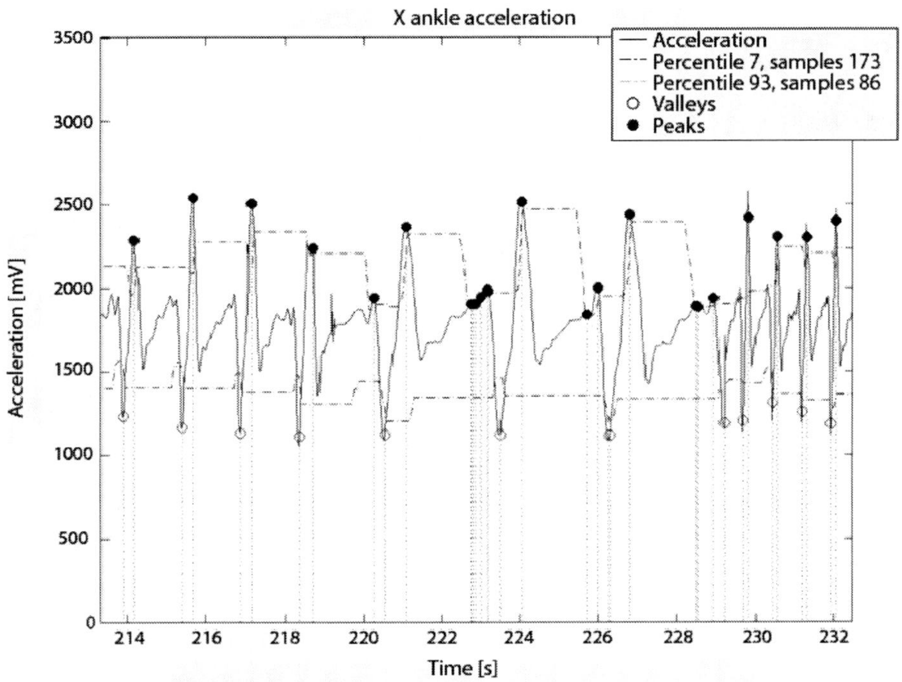

Figure 13. Adaptive response of the SGEDA to frequency modulation. Adapted from Torrealba R. R., Cappelletto J., Fermín L., Grieco J. C. & Fernández-López G. (2010): Statistics-based technique for automated detection of gait events from accelerometer signals. Electronics Letters, Vol. 46, No. 22, pp. 1483-1485.

5. Going Beyond Current Control Strategies

In practical terms, what gave applicable results in first commercial intelligent knee prostheses was 'soft control', using kinematic and kinetic signals captured in different points near the knee, mainly on the amputated leg. In fact, there was a real continuity in that development since the work of Bar et al. [61], following with the one of Aeyels et al. [62], until reaching the one of Herr and Wilkenfeld [19], which supported the commercially known Rheo Knee® [51]. Such prostheses were able to replace a natural knee joint on a human body, allowing the amputee to recover an acceptable human gait. Nonetheless, we still considered that that architecture limits the adaptive capability of electronically-controlled knee prostheses because it applies control by stages, unlike biological control, which is continuous. Therefore, we were interested in exploring the possibility of providing more natural biological control with this project. Two intelligent control strategies of this kind were approached. First, a control via central pattern generator (CPG), which was motivated by the biological process that generates the coordinated movements of legs observed in animal locomotion. This had been used for controlling biped robots [47, 63], but not for controlling a human prosthesis in the way we presented. Second, a continuous adaptive control (CAC) based on a gait speed dependent algorithm for setting an auto-adaptive proportional gain in the controller was employed. Gait speed was estimated using only the accelerometry data of the prosthetic leg, whereas the control action was applied on the knee axis through the prosthesis actuator.

5.1. CPG Approach

Regarding the first strategy, there were found several bio-inspired applications in robotics on locomotion of legged robots [47, 64]. In such sense, we asked the question, what if a reference of knee angle is generated to be followed by the prosthesis? The answer was found in central pattern generators (CPGs), which had been broadly used in the last decade to generate and coordinate motion of legs in walking robots, for executing all gait modes physically possible [65, 66]. Of course, there is a difference because the prosthesis is not a robotic device, designed to behave according to the programmer's orders but to the patient's will. However, technically, it is a matter of coupling the reference generated by the CPG with the prosthesis during walking, almost exactly what controllers do to enable robots to walk [67]. With this purpose in mind, a particular CPG was developed, based on Amplitude-Controlled Phase Oscillators (ACPOs) [68], and inserted in the control scheme as shown in Figure 14.

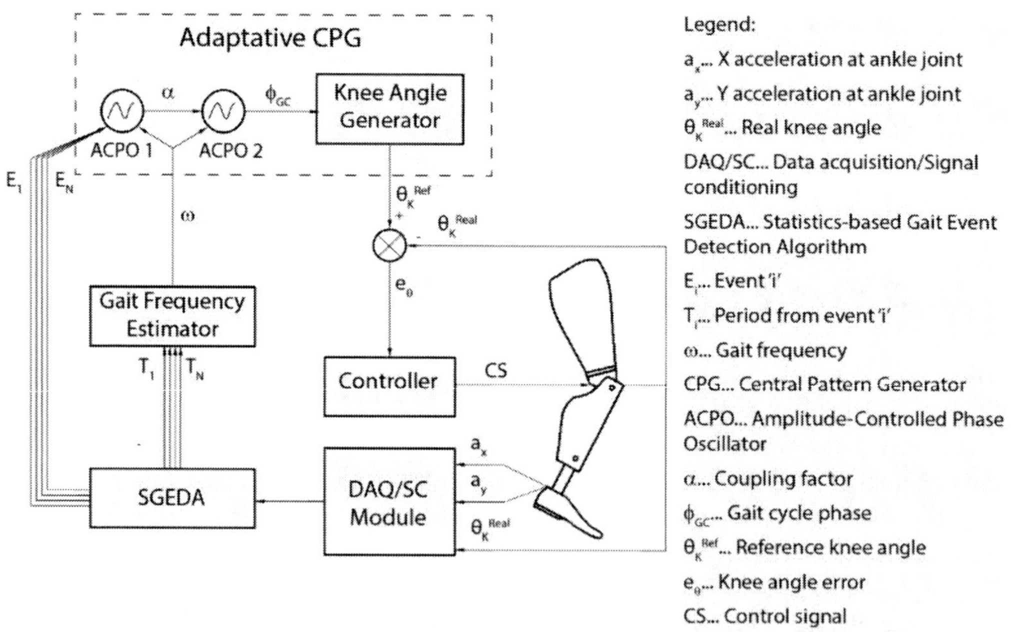

Figure 14. Control scheme of the knee prosthesis showing the ACPOs-based CPG. Adapted from Torrealba R. R., Cappelletto J., Fermín L., Fernández-López G. & Grieco J. C. (2012): Cybernetic knee prosthesis: application of an adaptive central pattern generator. Kybernetes: The International Journal of Systems & Cybernetics, Vol. 41, No. 1/2, pp. 192-205.

5.1.1. Control Scheme with Adaptive CPG

The CPG consisted of a couple of ACPOs unidirectionally connected and a knee angle generator (KAG) [69]. The ACPO 1 received the gait cycle events detected by the SGEDA, besides the gait frequency ω estimated from the corresponding gait periods of such events. The ACPO 2 received the ACPO 1 output through a coupling factor α and the frequency ω which was common to both oscillators.

The ACPO 2 output was a tracker signal ϕ_{GC}, which indicated the point that was running along the gait cycle from 0 to 100 per cent, obtained from its vector phase which ranged from 0 to 2Π. This was done in a continuous and smooth way, as the ACPOs worked solving differential equations for generating phase oscillations with controlled amplitude. The ϕ_{GC} went into the KAG, which in this case was developed as a simple interpolator that matched the current phase ϕ_{GC} with the corresponding angle of a sound knee along the gait cycle. In other words, the ACPOs tracked the gait cycle phase running on the prosthesis and the KAG generated the knee angle reference to be followed in order to mimic a natural gait.

5.1.2. Coupling of the CPG

In order to couple the CPG to the prosthesis, it is necessary to synchronize the oscillators with the real gait. It requires the detection of at least one singular event along the gait cycle, so every time this event occurs during walking, the ACPOs are synchronized by updating their phases. The more events are detected, the more accurate the CPG is, since its output frequency is set by the time between these events. For instance, if the gait cycle start is being detected [6, 70], the gait speed can be obtained from the period of this event, which is a measure of the gait frequency. This is the frequency used as reference input for the CPG frequency ω. However, if the gait speed changes during a gait cycle, then the CPG will not be updated until the next gait cycle starts, making the CPG very inaccurate. Furthermore, considering that the signal generated by the CPG would be used for controlling a prosthetic knee, an inaccurate output could mean the falling of the amputee user during walking. This is why detecting as many events as possible along gait cycle is mainly important, and must be taken into account when coupling the CPG to the real gait running in the prosthesis. In this regard, as aforementioned, the CPG coupling was performed through two ACPOs. The first ACPO updated its phase with every detected event, however, to avoid discontinuous changes in the CPG output, this ACPO was then connected to a second ACPO which produced the actual CPG phase reference. Such connection was done through a coupling factor α which set how hard the second ACPO would try to meet the reference of the first one. In other words, the first ACPO was hard-coupled with the gait on the prosthesis, and the second ACPO was soft-coupled with it.

5.1.3. Testing of the CPG Coupling

To test this approach, three kinds of trials were performed. The first set of trials was done with a healthy subject with both sound legs walking on a treadmill. The second set of trials was performed with this subject wearing the prosthesis being developed by the MRG by means of a special custom-made socket as shown in Figure 15, and finally, a third set of trials was carried out by a transfemoral amputee walking with this prosthesis on the treadmill as well, as seen in Figure 16b after adapting the prosthesis length as in Figure 16a.

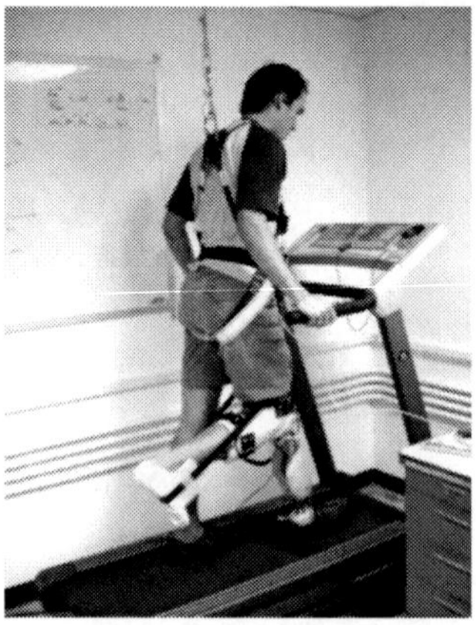

Figure 15. Subject with both sound legs walking with the prosthesis on the treadmill. Taken from Torrealba R. R., Cappelletto J., Fermín L., Fernández-López G. & Grieco J. C. (2012): Cybernetic knee prosthesis: application of an adaptive central pattern generator. Kybernetes: The International Journal of Systems & Cybernetics, Vol. 41, No. 1/2, pp. 192-205.

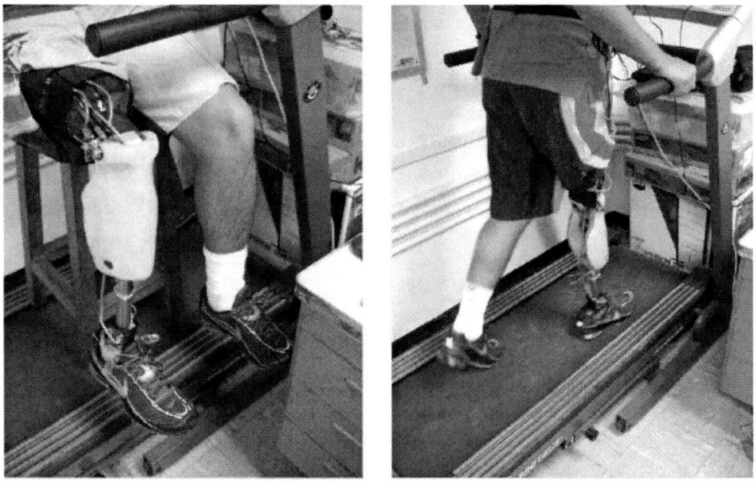

(a) (b)

Figure 16. Transfemoral amputee wearing the prosthesis: (a) Adjustment of the length, (b) Walking on the treadmill. Taken from Torrealba R. R., Pérez-D'Arpino C., Cappelletto J., Fermín-León L., Fernández-López G. & Grieco J. C. (2010): Through the development of a biomechatronic knee prosthesis for transfemoral amputees: mechanical design and manufacture, human gait characterization, intelligent control strategies and tests. IEEE Proceedings, International Conference on Robotics and Automation ICRA'2010, May 3-8, Anchorage, Alaska, USA, pp. 2934-2939.

5.1.3.1. Sound Leg Trials

These trials were performed with a healthy person walking on a level treadmill. During the trials, the subject was equipped with a bi-axial accelerometer and a knee articulated-support on one of his legs, and the data acquisition board placed on his back. The accelerometer (MMA7260Q, Freescale, USA) was placed at the ankle joint, specifically at the malleollus height, in such a way that the 'y'-axis went along the tibia and the 'x'-axis went perpendicular to it. The knee articulated-support was conditioned with a 5 KΩ potentiometer to capture the knee angle. These trials were performed at a constant speed of 2 kph set on the treadmill and all signals were captured and processed at a 60 Hz frequency. According to [56], it had been possible to detect the heel contact and toe-off events from this data. However, for the sake of simplicity, the CPG was synchronized using only the toe-off event, so every time it happened, the input ACPO phase was set to the respective percentage of gait cycle and restarted its oscillation. In particular, this event was detected by using only the 'x' acceleration, and the corresponding percentage of gait cycle was 60. These trials aimed to prove the detection of the toe-off event, showing the coupling of the CPG along the gait and generating the knee angle reference to be followed by the prosthesis.

5.1.3.2. Simulated Leg Trials

The first trials with the prosthesis were performed with the same subject used before; thus, a particular socket was designed to enable this subject to walk with the knee prosthesis, despite he was not an amputee. The reason for this was to get the system rightly tuned, before bringing a real patient to get involved with the trials at the lab. In particular, the socket resulted in such a way the subject introduced his right leg with the knee flexed at 90° and the prosthesis was aligned with the thigh in extended position as shown in Figure 15. Regarding the instrumentation, the knee prosthesis was equipped with a goniometer placed at the knee axis and a bi-axial accelerometer (MMA7260Q, Freescale, USA) placed at the ankle height. From these sensors, several events are detected [56], but again, for the sake of simplicity, only the toe-off event was taken into account. As before, this event was detected in real-time from the 'x' accelerometer data, and the knee angle reference was generated on-line by the CPG. Additionally, making use of the prosthesis goniometer, the real knee angle achieved with the prosthesis was measured and compared to the one generated by the CPG along the trial.

The first trials were carried out varying gait speed from 2 to 3 kph and then, from 3 to 2 kph again. Figure 17 shows the results corresponding to the increase of gait speed, while Figure 18 shows the corresponding ones to the decrease of gait speed. Both figures consist of the same four plots: the 'x' acceleration at ankle joint and the toe-off event detection, the ACPO 1 output, the ACPO 2 output, and the two knee angles, the real one and the CPG-generated.

From the first plot of Figure 17, it was observed that 'x' acceleration at ankle joint of the prosthetic leg was slightly different to the one of the sound leg. However, the toe-off event was detectable applying the same SGEDA used on the sound leg, although some omissions could occur, as it was the case on the third gait cycle of this trial. The second plot showed the ACPO 1 output. In this plot, it is clearly evident the robustness provided by the ACPO to the event detection algorithm.

Despite the aforesaid toe-off omission, the ACPO continued oscillating at its previous frequency and so, generating the gait cycle phase. Then, once the gait speed began to increase, it was also easily observable how the ACPO phase was moved forward, with the toe-off event occurring on the first plot and finally, it was stabilized again, once the gait speed reached a new constant value. Regarding the third plot, it allowed to see how the abrupt changes on the ACPO 1 were transformed in smooth changes through the ACPO 2, without losing the coupling with real gait. At last, the fourth plot showed several features to remark.

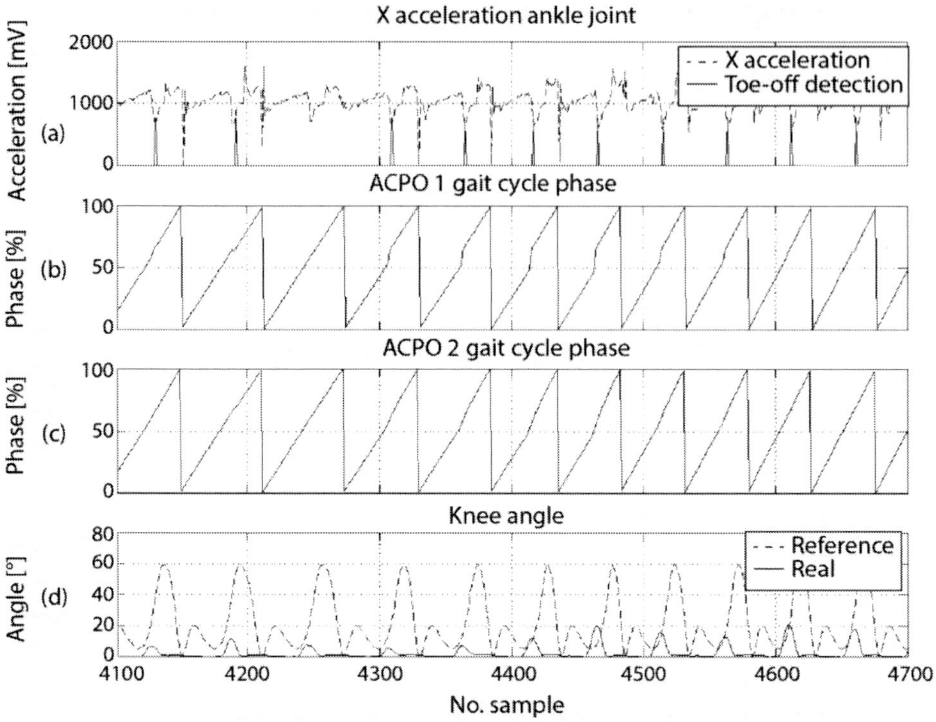

Figure 17. Results of the trial increasing gait speed from 2 to 3 kph on the treadmill. Adapted from Torrealba R. R., Cappelletto J., Fermín L., Fernández-López G. & Grieco J. C. (2012): Cybernetic knee prosthesis: application of an adaptive central pattern generator. Kybernetes: The International Journal of Systems & Cybernetics, Vol. 41, No. 1/2, pp. 192-205.

The first feature refers to the match between both knee angles, the real one and the CPG-generated. In this plot, it is shown how the real knee angle moves forward due to the gait speed increase, and it takes near four gait cycles to the CPG-generated knee angle to recover its synchronization with the first. The other feature regards the lower flexion angle reached by the prosthesis compared to a natural leg. On one hand, it was attributed to the fact that in this case, the knee prosthesis axis height was at least 10 cm lower than the corresponding one according to the subject's height, as this subject had its own sound knee. This definitely modified the natural gait biomechanics of the subject, and as a consequence, the knee angle of the prosthesis during walking. And on the other hand, it was also attributed to the fact that no control was being applied, and the prosthesis actuator took the knee to extension, once the toe-off occurred. However, as third feature, it was observed that this reduced knee flexion angle grew with gait speed. It went from 7 to 18° approximately, when going from 2 to 3 kph in this trial. Finally, the fourth feature observed was that the knee flexed only one time along the gait cycle, whereas two times is the natural. A first flexion should occur after heel contact, when the leg is loaded by the body moving forward, and the knee flexes to decelerate and absorb the impact. Then, the knee should go to extension again, before the second flexion begins. The second flexion corresponds to pre-swing during the stance phase, which was the one actually occurring, as shown in the fourth plot of Figure 17. As observed, the knee was completely extended during the stance phase until pre-swing. This is typical in knee prosthesis users to protect themselves from a fall. They block the knee by extending the hip during the first stages of stance phase, as otherwise the knee buckles and hence, they fall.

The results presented in Figure 18 are similar to the ones of Figure 17, but reducing the gait speed. In both cases, the need of coupling the CPG with the real gait becomes evident, otherwise the virtual reference gets lost and never recovers the synchronization with the actual knee angle reference required at the joint. Likewise, it is important to remark the fact that, although the CPG coupling was done from the toe-off detection, which resulted an abrupt correction of the ACPO 1 gait phase as shown in the second plot, the final behavior of the CPG, when faced to speed changes, was smoothed by the ACPO 2 as observed in the third plot of Figure 18. This is explained by the way in which the ACPOs work, and how they were coupled, which turns even an abrupt input as a delta, in a smooth and continuous response. Regarding the fourth plot, it is interesting to see how in this case, the real knee angle begins to move backwards due to the deceleration, and how the CPG copes with this change to recover the coupling with the actual gait.

5.1.3.3. Prosthetic Leg Trials

The last trials were performed with an amputee patient walking with the prosthesis at 2.5 kph on the treadmill. The results are shown in Figure 19, which consists of two plots. The first plot is the 'x' acceleration captured at ankle height on the prosthetic leg, as well as the toe-off detection carried out with the same algorithm used so far.

The second plot shows both knee angles, the real one captured on the prosthesis and the virtual one generated by the CPG. From the first plot, it is observed that some toe-offs were not detected; however, as the CPG was already coupled with the gait and the speed was not changing, the CPG continued oscillating and resumed its coupling with the next event detection. But what if gait speed changes when toe-off event is not detected? In this case, the CPG will get lost until at least two continuous events are detected, which will allow to calculate the new gait period and update it. Nevertheless, if gait speed keeps changing, it will take too long to the CPG, to actually meet the real gait by detecting just one event per gait cycle. This is why the detection of as many events as possible along a gait cycle is important, since every event detected allows to update the CPG phase, enabling a faster coupling with the real gait. Regarding the second plot, the first feature that came out was the fact that the knee angle reached with the prosthesis being used by an amputee was considerably higher than the one reached when the prosthesis was used by the subject with sound legs. This confirmed the aforementioned hypothesis regarding the lower knee flexion angle observed in the last case.

It is also shown the synchronization between the real knee angle and the generated from the CPG, which demonstrated again the feasibility of coupling it to the actual gait on the prosthesis, this time in real conditions as it was being used by a transfemoral amputee. Finally, the blocking of the knee during the first stages of the stance phase was observed again. As mentioned before, this results natural in prosthesis user amputees to avoid the knee buckling and thus, a potential fall.

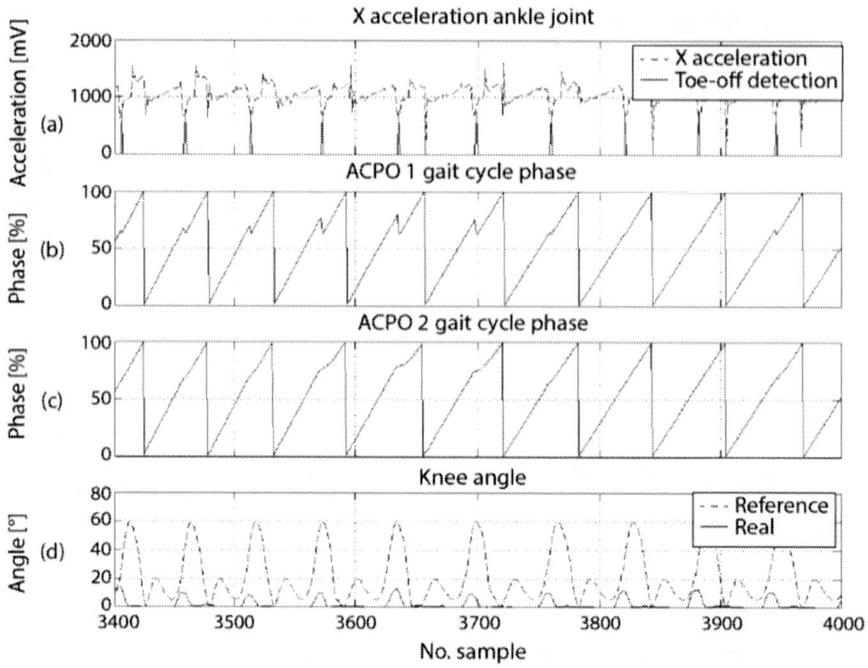

Figure 18. Results of the trial decreasing gait speed from 3 to 2 kph on the treadmill. Adapted from Torrealba R. R., Cappelletto J., Fermín L., Fernández-López G. & Grieco J. C. (2012): Cybernetic knee prosthesis: application of an adaptive central pattern generator. Kybernetes: The International Journal of Systems & Cybernetics, Vol. 41, No. 1/2, pp. 192-205.

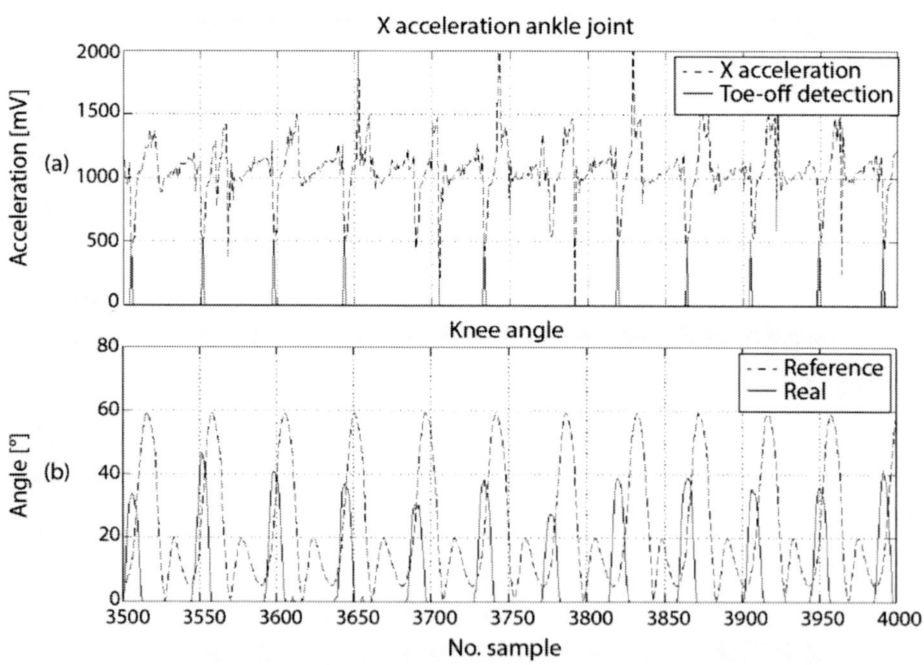

Figure 19. Test results of control with reference knee angle via CPG. Adapted from Torrealba R. R., Cappelletto J., Fermín L., Fernández-López G. & Grieco J. C. (2012): Cybernetic knee prosthesis: application of an adaptive central pattern generator. Kybernetes: The International Journal of Systems & Cybernetics, Vol. 41, No. 1/2, pp. 192-205.

On the prosthesis performance using the CPG, two flaws were found. The first flaw was that the actuator took the prosthesis to extension once the foot was off the floor. Thus, no further flexion was possible during swing and therefore, the natural maximum knee angle of 60° was impossible with this prosthesis as observed from Figure 19b. Nevertheless, the patient remarked that the prosthesis must return to extension as fast as possible during swing, so it is completely straight before next heel contact. Tests with more individuals were required to determine the real impact of this limitation on the prosthesis performance.

The second flaw was that the amplitude of knee angle is directly proportional to gait speed. However, given the first drawback, it was never approached though it is solvable by simply modulating the amplitude of the knee angle reference with gait speed.

5.2. CAC Approach

The rest of the control scheme shown in Figure 14 referring the generation of a control signal for the prosthesis was never developed with the CPG approach. Indeed, from the analysis of the CPG strategy results previously presented, the idea of making the prosthesis to follow a reference generated by a CPG was discarded as long as the prosthesis is equipped with that MR actuator; moreover, we realized that the control action should not be only attached to the gait cycle but also to the knee angle directly. Consequently, the second strategy applied a proportional control action directly coupled to the knee angle measured on the prosthesis. In this sense, a control signal was conceived to be applied after the maximum knee angle reached by the prosthesis at toe-off, allowing the knee to flex freely during terminal stance and pre-swing, and later to extend in a dampened way according to gait period during the swing phase, guaranteeing complete extension before next heel strike. Also, we insisted in achieving a natural flexion of the knee during load response sub-phase by applying a control signal in a form of a dampened step. Such scheme results adaptive because it attaches the control action to the gait period through a parameter defined as 'settling time', which is the time it takes the knee to full-extend during swing phase. This feature allowed to disregard characterization of gait cycle as done so far, as the control action was directly coupled to the prosthesis knee angle; barely detection of gait cycle events is required to calculate gait period from which control action is modulated.

5.2.1. General Scheme of Continuous Adaptive Controller

The scheme control is presented in Figure 20. As seen, there was a data acquisition and signal conditioning module that received knee and ankle accelerations plus the knee angle. Once conveniently-filtered, these signals were sent as input to the SGEDA, which as before, utilized auto-adaptive thresholds to detect particular features on these considered as gait events. The SGEDA computed a gait period T_i for every gait event detected and then, these were sent to the gait period estimator (GPE) which set the current gait period T^*. Every period T_i referred to the number of samples that passed between the occurrence of a couple of consecutives events 'i', as the GPE had an input for every event 'i' detected. Subsequently, for making the controller adapts to gait speed changes, the gait period T^* went into the continuous adaptive controller (CAC), which was actually composed by two controllers: one for the stance phase and the other for the swing phase.

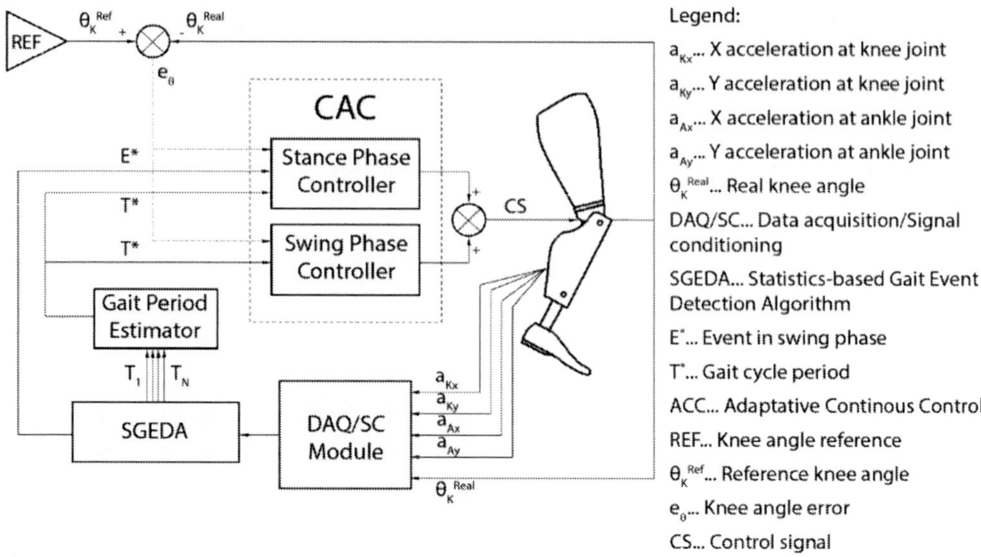

Figure 20. Control scheme of the knee prosthesis showing the CAC.

Both controllers received the gait period T* as input, while the stance phase controller received the event E* in addition. The latter triggered its control action and was identified from one of the accelerations captured at the knee height on the prosthesis. On the other hand, the swing phase controller only acted during extension of the prosthesis on air, so its triggering event may be deemed as the maximum flexion angle reached by the prosthesis at toe-off. The real knee angle θ_K^{Real} measured on the prosthesis was compared with a pre-defined reference θ_K^{Ref} and the difference between both e_θ was fed to both stance and swing phase controllers of the CAC. Finally, outputs of these controllers were added to obtain the control signal that was sent to the prosthesis actuator.

5.2.2. Scheme of Swing Phase Adaptive Proportional Controller

More in detail, the swing phase controller (SwC) is presented in Figure 21. As seen, a reference settling time t_{ST}^{Ref} of the prosthesis was defined from the gait period T* as a value proportional to this. On the other hand, the real settling time t_{ST}^{Real} was measured by the SGEDA from the knee angle signal θ_K^{Real}. Then, both settling times were compared yielding an error e_t^{ST} which went into the SwC. Inside this controller, a factor F_c generated a difference ΔK_p proportional to the error e_t^{ST}. Such difference updated the proportional constant K_p of the controller by adding the new ΔK_p to the current K_p corresponding to the previous gait cycle. Finally, this updated K_p multiplied by the knee angle difference e_θ, obtained from knee reference angle θ_K^{Ref} and the knee real one θ_K^{Real}, was the swing control signal (SwCS). Thus, this SwC resulted a self-tuning regulator (STR) controller in which the settling time is the 'behavior parameter' that allows to adjust the gain K_p automatically (auto-tuning) by the integrator effect utilized to correct the error e_t^{ST} that goes into the controller.

According to the aforementioned, the proportional gain K_p is adapted to the user's gait speed. If it increases, the K_p is reduced in order to allow the knee to extend rapidly and conversely, if gait speed is decreased, then the K_p is augmented in order to slow knee extension. The gait speed is estimated through the events detected by the SGEDA.

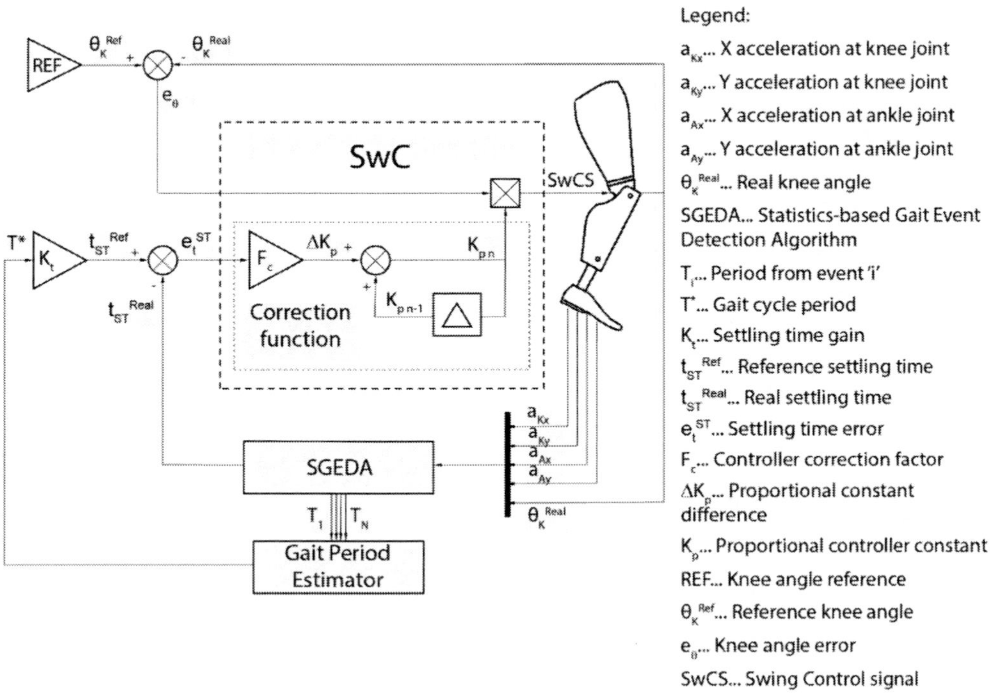

Figure 21. Control scheme of the knee prosthesis showing the STR-based SwC.

No other characterization of the gait cycle is required. In order to cope with possible false detections, two different measures were taken: a median filter applied to the different gait period estimations obtained from each pair of equivalent events, and the other measure was to take into account that a singular event (heel contact, for example) cannot occur two or more consecutive times in one gait cycle. For this, it was developed a logical filter to remove consecutive repeated detections.

5.2.3. Testing of the CAC Performance

To test the prosthesis performance under this approach, the previous volunteer was invited again. After adjusting the prosthesis to his height as seen in Figure 16a, several trials were performed with him walking on the treadmill while applying the novel CAC described above on the prosthesis. Special emphasis was put on gait speed changes particularly to verify the CAC adaptability. In this regard, before analyzing results presented in Figure 22, it is worthy to mention that though it has been said that control action is coupled to knee angle in this approach, it is a soft-coupling, as the final SwC signal comes from the STR control loop. As a matter of fact, there was observed a delay between gait speed and the proportional gain K_p. For example, when the gait speed decreased, as in 45.7s (see Figure 22a), the K_p began to increase after two gait cycles (see Figure 22b).

Then, for a gait speed increase, as in 57s, the K_p decreased after one gait cycle, as observed at 58s. Those delays are not symmetrical in time duration. Such asymmetry occurs because the estimation of walking speed was obtained each time an event was detected, thus at a low gait speed, the update rate was lower than at a higher gait speed.

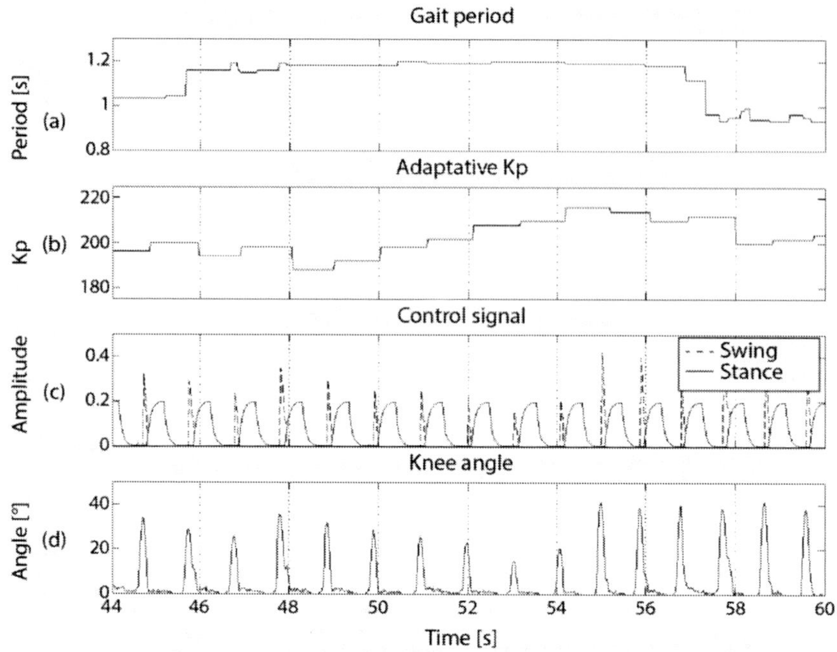

Figure 22. Test results of CAC with non-characterized gait cycle. Adapted from Torrealba R. R., Pérez-D'Arpino C., Cappelletto J., Fermín-León L., Fernández-López G. & Grieco J. C. (2010): Through the development of a biomechatronic knee prosthesis for transfemoral amputees: mechanical design and manufacture, human gait characterization, intelligent control strategies and tests. IEEE Proceedings, International Conference on Robotics and Automation ICRA'2010, May 3-8, Anchorage, Alaska, USA, pp. 2934-2939.

In Figure 22c, both control signals are shown: a step signal corresponding to the stance phase, and the proportional signal that follows the knee angle, but applies only during extension in the swing phase. The control signal corresponding to the stance phase was included, to avoid the knee buckling during load response after heel contact. Finally, Figure 22d shows the knee angle achieved with the CAC strategy and the prosthesis worn by a transfemoral amputee. This approach resulted in a simple and effective means for controlling the prosthesis designed in this project. This removed the need for characterizing the gait cycle in terms of specific events and also allowed for dealing with the change of knee angle amplitude as a function of gait speed because the control action is directly coupled to the joint axis.

6. Evolving from Passive to Active through a New Compliant Actuator

6.1. Mechanism Optimization

Although this first prototype complied with all the structural requirements, as this supported the patient weight and floor reaction loads applied on the prosthesis during walking, it must be pointed out that the knee prosthesis weight was above the one of its commercial counterparts. On the other hand, the manufacturing process of the chassis was mostly manual, resulting time-consuming and little precise. By then, those concluding remarks brought out the need of carrying out a redesign of this first prototype to attend these drawbacks.

First, a new design for the chassis was proposed, separating the structural part from the aesthetic one, i.e., a mechanism consisting of a metallic frame was introduced to support the loads, while a plastic cosmetic cover fits on it to provide the prosthesis with a natural human leg appearance. The mechanism was designed to be made of aluminum with its axes made of stainless steel; the cover would be 3D printed in ABS. Later, a structural optimization of the mechanism was performed applying stress analysis via Finite Element Method (FEM), a well-proved structural mechanics approach [71,72]. This process was done with ANSYS® Workbench 10.0 working interconnected with ProENGINEER® Wildfire 3.0. It was very useful because according to the loads and boundary conditions indicated by the ISO10328 [48], as well as the materials involved, it showed where to remove material because it was not needed to support loads, and where to keep it because otherwise the part would experience failure. As result, an optimized monocentric knee mechanism including its chassis was obtained as shown in Figure 23, yielding an approximate weight of 1,691 g including the commercial MR actuator. This represented a reasonable weight reduction of 21.8% regarding the former prototype, and specifically, regarding the chassis, it went up to 41% in weight reduction.

These outcomes were remarkable towards the ultimate goal of the project, which is the development of an intelligent knee prosthesis feasible of manufacturing on an assembly line and also, competitive before other commercial equivalent prostheses. Should the lector look for further details on this point, please go to [73].

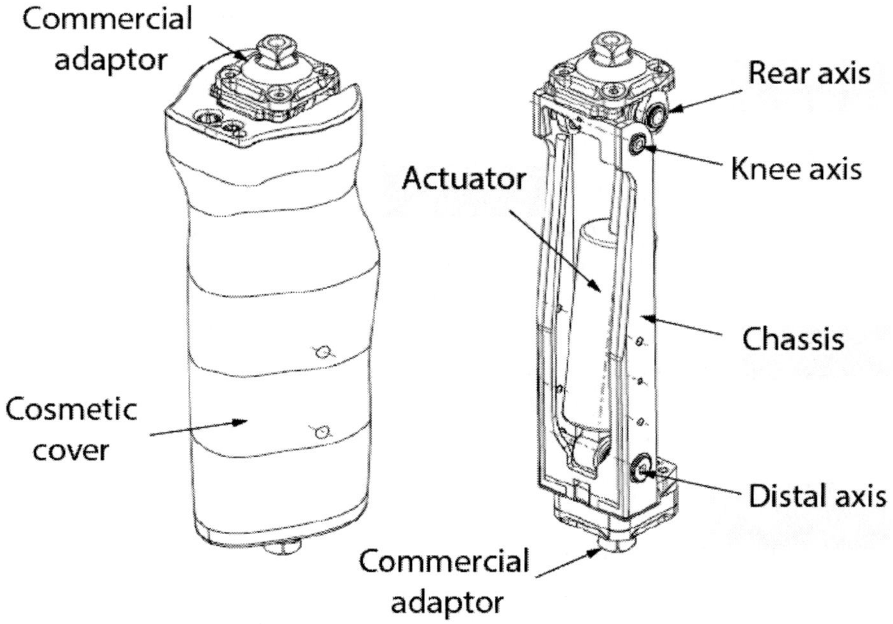

Figure 23. Resulting knee mechanism optimized via FEM to reduce weight.

6.2. Exoskeleton Actuator Transitivity

More recently, in 2013, also included in the DODT research line of the MRG, a new project was begun having the purpose of developing an exoskeleton for human gait rehabilitation. By that moment, one of the first requirements that jumped on the drawing table were the joint actuators to be utilized. Once again, eyes were turned to robotics having variable impedance actuators (VIAs) on the sight this time. VIAs, a.k.a. compliant or variable stiffness actuators, result from the need of robotics to create human-friendly robots capable of interaction with humans and other robots in a safe manner. This regards especially to dealing with collisions, and also, to an efficient use of the energy through modulation of the position-stiffness response of the actuators at the joints [74-78].

6.2.1. Design of a Variable Impedance Actuator for Knee Joint

Afterwards, taking advantage of the know-how acquired with the development of the intelligent knee prosthesis presented before in this chapter, we decided to start by creating an actuator for the knee joint of the exoskeleton. An exoskeleton may be considered an orthosis, so on one hand, there will be an interaction with the real leg of the user, which is not presented in the case of the prosthesis, but on the other one, considering an exoskeleton with rehabilitation purposes, requirements would be (at the most) the same of the prosthesis, which has to completely carry with the loads associated to the loss limb during walking. In particular, the maximum torque of knee joint along gait cycle was taken as the maximum nominal torque required from the actuator in case this would have to completely assume the load for moving the knee joint, for example during the first stages of rehabilitation of a severe impaired patient. Regarding the knee angle, a range from 0-90° for including sitting-standing transitions was also established. And finally, considering the knee angular velocity and torque during walking, it was obtained the maximum power demanded at the knee joint. Taking all this into account, design criteria for the knee actuator were established.

Bearing in mind these design criteria, a broad review of the state-of-the-art of VIAs was performed. From this, the FSJ (Floating Spring Joint) [74] and BAVS (Bidirectional Antagonistic Variable Stiffness) [78,79], models emerged as the most suitable designs. The FSJ design introduces a floating spring to exert a pulling force on a pair of cam disks that embrace the cam rollers. The relative motion of the cam disks over the cam rollers results in a passive deflection of the joint and thus, adjusting the stiffness of the actuator is done by controlling such relative motion through a particular electrical motor dedicated to this task, which is significantly smaller than the other one dedicated to control the joint position. For the MRG design, however, both of the electrical motors selected had the same size and relative low power compared to the one used by the FSJ as joint motor. This situation turned the design towards the BAVS approach in which there are two motors of same size adding their torques at the output of the actuator; therefore, it was decided to combine both designs in a new one called BAFSA (Bidirectional Antagonistic Floating Spring Actuator).

6.2.2. Details and Functioning of the BAFSA

BAFSA is characterized for its cam shape. Cam shape could be made from a simple spline or mathematical function, nevertheless we did a special effort onto the design of such geometry for maximizing variability of stiffness. Though particular details of such design are out of the scope of this chapter, it must be pointed out that an optimal geometry for the cam was obtained using cubic Bézier curves and a differential evolution algorithm with a cost function expressed in terms of the torque produced by the actuator. Readers interested in a further insight into this design can find a particularly dedicated paper in [80]. Regarding the mechanism, it consists of two electrical motors of same size each connected to a shaft through a couple of gears. These gears are aligned with the axis of the mechanism and are located at the opposed ends of the actuator as shown in Figure 24.

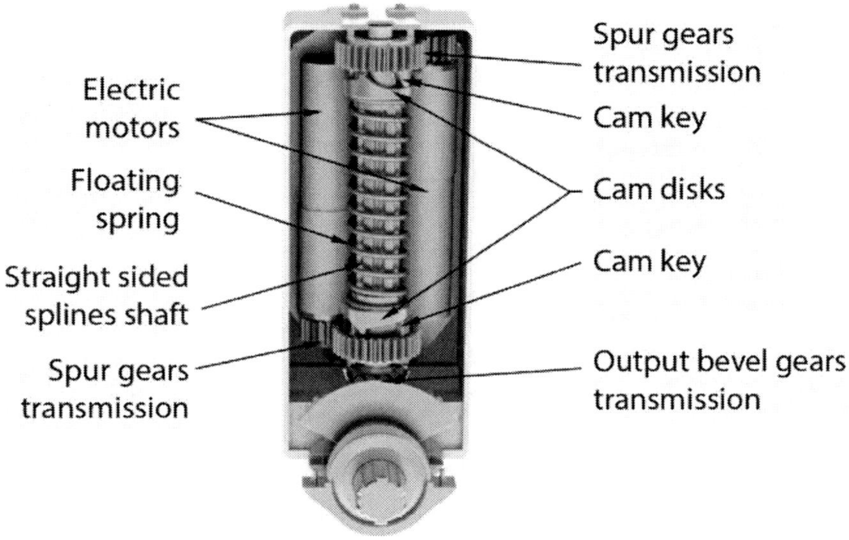

Figure 24. Mechanism of the BAFSA.

The cam rollers are attached to the shaft and exert a force (through the cam key) on the cam disks located at both ends of the floating spring. Both cam disks are attached to a frame that holds a pinion bevel gear which is the output of the BAFSA. However, the complete actuator for the exoskeleton at the knee joint also includes the speed reduction incorporated by the transmission between the bevel pinion and its crown (see Figure 24), which is the one that finally increase the output torque of the actuator up to the maximum expected.

Motors can rotate in the same or opposite directions. Being counter-mounted, when they rotate in the same direction, it actually means that the cam rollers rotate in opposed directions and it turns out a compression of the spring as the cam rollers spin on the steep surface of cam disks. Indeed, this spring loading is the way to modulate the actuator response in terms of stiffness: the higher the spring compression, the higher the stiffness offered by the actuator before external forces.

This configuration is called 'normal mode', the other one consisting in rotating the motors in opposed directions is called 'helping mode'. In this case, both cam rollers rotate in the same direction moving the cam disks as well. Finally, such rotation is transmitted to the frame and from there to the joint through the couple of bevel gears. This is the way in which the actuator operates to modulate the angular position of the joint.

6.2.3. Embedding the BAFSA into the Intelligent Knee Prosthesis

Though the BAFSA was originally conceived to work as the actuator of the knee joint on the exoskeleton, once it was designed, we came up with the idea of adapting it to the chassis of the knee prosthesis we have initially created. Such adaptation did not take much more than the work already done. As a matter of fact, from the mechanism shown in Figure 23, minor changes were performed on the chassis to hold the new actuator. The complete prosthesis equipped with the BAFSA inside is shown in Figure 25.

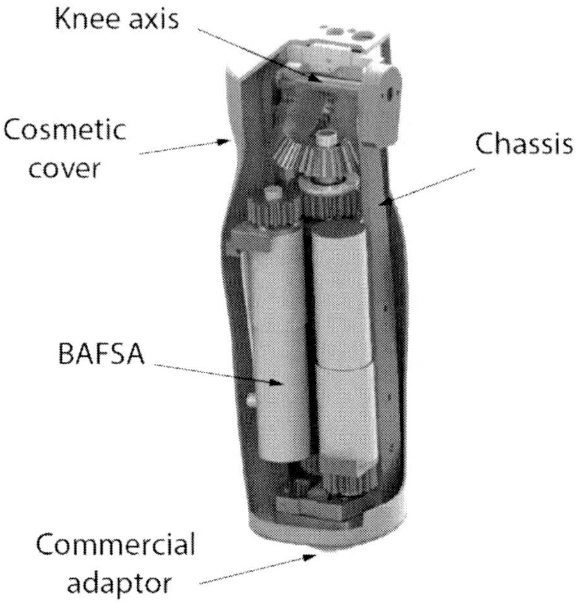

Figure 25. External intelligent knee prosthesis equipped with the BAFSA (knee joint suppressed of the assembly to ease view of the BAFSA embedded).

By doing this adaptation, we would be taking our intelligent knee prosthesis from passive to active through a novel compliant actuator. As aforementioned, the requirements considered to design the BAFSA were the same ones deemed for designing the knee prosthesis, therefore, it should work well as actuator of the intelligent knee prosthesis we created first. Furthermore, in this case, control is simpler than on the exoskeleton as there is no interaction with the level of impairment of the patient treated. Future developments on the control strategy to be applied on the BAFSA to render the best biomimicked behavior of a sound leg with the knee prosthesis are going to be required. However, all the advances presented in this chapter regarding the development of the passive intelligent knee prosthesis will be put on practice on the active one. In this sense, instrumentation and subsequent characterization of gait cycle is already done. And on the other hand, CPG approach presented here will be surely resumed, probably mixed somehow with the CAC strategy also outlined before, but having this time an enhanced ability in terms of the versatility achieved through the position-stiffness relationship offered by the BAFSA at the knee axis.

Conclusion

This chapter has presented an extended summary of the evolution experienced in the development of an external intelligent knee prosthesis. In fact, this has not only outlined the technical aspects involved, but also has covered most of them providing a detailed insight. A complex and multi-disciplinary project as this must entail several topics in order to accomplish its final goal. In this case, a complete review and subsequent innovation on the state-of-the-art encountered has been presented regarding knee prostheses mechanisms, instrumentation and techniques utilized to characterize gait cycle, theoretical and practical control strategies proposed and tested on prototypes and commercial intelligent prosthetic knees, and finally, actuators technologies used on the quest for mimicking the always-best-example of nature; this time referring the biomechanical behavior of a sound knee. This chapter has been a unique opportunity for us to organize and present all the work done so far in this endeavor of creating an external intelligent knee prosthesis for transfemoral amputees. Likewise, we are proud of having shown advances on the field and with them, having done creative contributions in this ever-growing universe of prosthetics and orthotics to improve quality of life of human beings with disabilities.

Acknowledgments

The authors gratefully acknowledge the contribution of C. P. O. Fernando Carvalho, for his assistance in the design and manufacture of the prosthesis chassis, as well to all the personnel of his workshop BIOTECPRO, C. A. Also, we are deeply grateful to Mr. Fernando Luzardo, for offering himself as volunteer to test the prosthesis during the development of this project.

This project was initially funded by the Project No. 195 through the Technological Park of Sartenejas in accordance with the Science, Technology and Innovation Law of Venezuela, and currently, it is being funded by the Project No. PEI-2147 of the National Fund for Science, Innovation and Technology of Venezuela.

Also, it has been sponsored by the Technological Park of Sartenejas, the Foundation for Research and Development, and the Deanship of Research and Development of the Simón Bolívar University.

References

[1] Ziegler-Graham, K., MacKenzie, E. J., Ephraim, P. L., Travison, T. G. & Brookmeyer, R. (2008). Estimating the prevalence of limb loss in the United States – 2005 to 2050. *Archives of Physical Medicine and Rehabilitation*, *Vol. 89*, *No. 3*, pp. 422-429.

[2] Barouti, H., Agnello, M. & Volckmann, P. (1998). Amputations du membre supérieur. *Kinésithérapie-Médecine Physique-Réadaptation*, *26-269-A-10*, pp. 1-11.

[3] Kirtley, C. *Clinical Gait Analysis Theory and Practice*. 1st Edition. Churchill Livingstone Elsevier; 2006.

[4] Flowers, W. & Mann, R. (1977). An electrohydraulic knee-torque controller for a prosthesis simulator. *ASME Transactions of the Journal of Biomechanical Engineering, No. 99*, pp. 3-8.

[5] Darling, D. Automatic damping profile optimization for computer controlled above-knee prostheses. Masters thesis. Boston, MA-USA: Massachusetts Institute of Technology, Department of Mechanical Engineering; 1978.

[6] Grimes, D. An active multi-mode above-knee prosthesis controller. Doctoral thesis. Boston, MA-USA: Massachusetts Institute of Technology, Department of Mechanical Engineering; 1979.

[7] Torrealba, R. R., Fernández-López, G. & Grieco, J. C. (2008). Towards the development of knee prostheses: review of current researches. *Kybernetes: The International Journal of Systems & Cybernetics, Vol. 37, No. 9/10*, pp. 1561-1576.

[8] Radcliffe, C. (1977). Above knee prosthetics. *Prosthetics and Orthotics International, No. 1*, pp. 146-160.

[9] Näder, M. & Näder, H. Otto Bock Prostheses Compendium: Prostheses for Lower Limbs. 2nd Edition. Berlin: Schiele & Schön GmbH; 1993.

[10] Endolite (2006): Above Knee Systems – Endolite North America – Lower Extremity Prosthetics [online]. Available from: www.endolite.com/ak.htm (accessed April 2, 2006).

[11] Otto Bock (2007): Otto Bock Microprocessor Knees. C-Leg – Otto Bock [online]. Available from: http://ottobockus.com/PRODUCTS/LOWER_LIMB_PROSTHETICS/c-leg.asp (accessed November 3, 2007).

[12] Rheo Knee (2007): Bionic Technology. Rheo knee – Ossur [online]. Available from: www.ossur.com/?pageid=2734 (accessed November 3, 2007).

[13] Staros, A. (1964). The principles of swing-phase control: the advantages of fluid mechanisms. *Prostheses, Braces and Technical Aids, No. 13*, pp. 11-16.

[14] Lewis, E. (1965). Fluid-control knee mechanisms: clinical considerations. *Bulletin of Prosthetics Research, No. 10*, pp. 24-56.

[15] Mauch, H. (1968). Stance control for above-knee artificial legs – design considerations in the S-N-S knee. *Bulletin of Prosthetics Research, No. 10*, pp. 61-72.

[16] Whittle, M. W. GAIT ANALYSIS AN INTRODUCTION. 4th Edition. BUTTERWORTH HEINEMANN ELSEVIER; 2007.

[17] Winter, D. A. Biomechanics and Motor Control of Human Movement. 4th Edition. Hoboken, New Jersey: John Wiley & Sons, Inc.; 2009.

[18] Blumentritt, S., Scherer, H., Michael, J. & Schmalz, T. (1998). Transfemoral amputees walking on a rotary hydraulic prosthetic knee mechanism: a preliminary report. *Journal of Prosthetics and Orthotics, Vol. 10, No. 3*, pp. 61-70 [online]. Available from: www.oandp.org/jpo/library/1998_03_061.asp (accessed February 8, 2006).

[19] Herr, H. & Wilkenfeld, A. (2003). User-adaptive control of a magnetorheological prosthetic knee. *Industrial Robot: An International Journal, Vol. 30, No. 1*, pp. 42-55.

[20] Stinus, H. (2000). Biomechanik und Beurteilung des mikroprozessorgesteurten Exoprothesenkniegelenkes C-Leg (Biomechanics and evaluation of the microprocessor-controlled C-Leg exoprosthesis knee joint). *Orthopädie Technik, Vol. 138, No. 3*, pp. 278-282.

[21] Murray, M., Mollinger, L., Sepic, S. & Gardner, G. (1983). Gait patterns in above-knee amputee patients: hydraulic swing control vs. constant-friction knee components. *Archives of Physical Medicine and Rehabilitation, No. 64*, pp. 339-345.

[22] Kastner, J., Nimmervoll, R., Kristen, H. & Wagner, P. (1999). What are the benefits of the C-Leg? A comparative gait analysis of the C-Leg, the 3R45 and the 3R80 prosthetic knee joints. *Medizinisch-Orthopädische Technik, No. 119*, pp. 131-137 [online]. Available from: http://ottobockus.com/products/lower_limb_prosthetics/c-leg_benefits.pdf (accessed January 25, 2006).

[23] Schmalz, T., Blumentritt, S. & Jarasch, R. (2002). A comparison of different prosthetic knee joints during step over step stair descent. *Orthopädie Technik, No. 7*, pp. 586-592 [online]. Available from: http://ottobockus.com/products/lower_limb_prosthetics/schmalz_joints.pdf (accessed January 25, 2006).

[24] Meier, M., Hansen, A. & Gard, S. (2005). Performance on an obstacle course: Otto Bock C-Leg vs. Otto Bock 3R60 vs. Catech SNS. 2005 Journal of Proceedings of the Microprocessor Knee Symposium of the American Academy of Orthotists and Prosthetists, pp. 5-8 [online]. Available from: www.oandp.org/publications/jop/2005/2005-5.asp (accessed February 8, 2006).

[25] Peeraer, L., Aeyels, B. & Van der Perre, G. (1990). Development of EMG-based mode and intent recognition algorithms for a computer-controlled above-knee prosthesis. *Journal of Biomedical Engineering, No. 12*, pp. 178-182.

[26] Schmalz, T., Blumentritt, S., Tsukishiro, K., Köcher, L. & Dietl, H. (1998). Energy efficiency of trans-femoral amputees walking on computer-controlled prosthetic knee joint C-Leg. Proceedings of the 9th World Congress of the International Society for Prosthetics and Orthotics, Amsterdam-The Netherlands, pp. 459-460 [online]. Available from: http://ottobockus.com/products/lower_limb_prosthetics/c-leg_energy.pdf (accessed January 25, 2006).

[27] Buckley, J., Spence, W. & Solomonidis, S. (1997). Energy cost of walking: comparison of intelligent prosthesis with conventional mechanism. *Archives of Physical Medicine and Rehabilitation, No. 78*, pp. 330-333.

[28] Johansson, J. L., Sherrill, D. M., Riley, P. O., Bonato, P. & Herr, H. (2005). A clinical comparison of variable-damping and mechanically passive prosthetic knee devices. *American Journal of Physical Medicine and Rehabilitation, Vol. 84, No. 8*, pp. 563-575.

[29] Elliott, S. (2005). Outcome assessment of a MR microprocessor-controlled knee. 2005 Journal of Proceedings of the Microprocessor Knee Symposium of the American Academy of Orthotists and Prosthetists, pp. 1-4 [online]. Available from: www.oandp.org/publications/jop/2005/2005-5.asp (accessed February 8, 2006).

[30] De Roy, K. (2005). Powered prosthetics: clinical outcome of unprecedented function. 2005 Journal of Proceedings of the Microprocessor Knee Symposium of the American Academy of Orthotists and Prosthetists, pp. 8-10 [online]. Available from: www.oandp.org/publications/jop/2005/2005-5.asp (accessed February 8, 2006).

[31] Zlatnik, D., Steiner, B. & Schweitzer, G. (2002). Finite-state control of a trans-femoral (TF) prosthesis. *IEEE Transactions on Control Systems Technology, Vol. 10, No. 3*, pp. 408-420.

[32] Gupta, B. & Anand, H. (2004). A step towards anthropomorphic prosthetic knee. Paper presentation contest at Effervescence IIITA, Allahabad-India, October 1-3, 2005.

[33] Jonic, S., Jankovic, T., Gajic, V. & Popovic, D. (1999). Three machine learning techniques for automatic determination of rules to control locomotion. *IEEE Transactions on Biomedical Engineering, Vol. 46, No. 3*, pp. 300-310.

[34] Popovic, M., Englehart, A. & Herr, H. (2004). Angular momentum primitives for human walking: biomechanics and control. Proceedings of the 2004 IEEE/RSJ International Conference on Intelligent Robots and Systems IROS'2004, Sendai-Japan, pp. 1685-1691.

[35] Kampas, P. (2001). The optimal use of myoelectrodes. Translation of: *Medizinisch-Orthopädische Technik, No. 121*, pp. 21-27.

[36] Fleischer, C. & Hommel, G. (2005). EMG-driven human model for orthosis control. Proceedings of the 6th International Workshop 'Human Interaction with Machines', Springer, Berlin, pp. 69-76.

[37] Shahid, S., Walker, J., Lyons, G., Byrne, C. & Vishwanath, A. (2005). Application of higher order statistics techniques to EMG signals to characterize the motor unit action potential. *IEEE Transactions on Biomedical Engineering, Vol. 52, No. 7*, pp. 1195-1209.

[38] Park, E. & Meek, S. (1993). Fatigue compensation of the electromyographic signal for prosthetics control and force estimation. *IEEE Transactions on Biomedical Engineering, Vol. 40, No. 10*, pp. 1019-1023.

[39] Hoover, C. D., Fulk, G. D. & Fite, K. B. (2013). Stair ascent with a powered transfemoral prosthesis under direct myoelectric control. *IEEE/ASME Transactions on Mechatronics, Vol. 18, No. 3*, pp. 1191-1200.

[40] Wu, S. K., Waycaster, G. & Shen, X. (2011). Electromyography-based control of active above-knee prostheses. *Control Engineering Practice, Vol. 19, No. 8*, pp. 875-882.

[41] Ha, K. H., Varol, H. A. & Goldfarb, M. (2011). Volitional control of a prosthetic knee using surface electromyography. *IEEE Transactions on Biomedical Engineering, Vol. 58, No. 1*, pp. 144–151.

[42] Brambilla, G., Buchli, J. & Ijspeert, A. (2006). Adaptive four legged locomotion control based on nonlinear dynamical systems. Proceedings of the 9th International Conference on the SIMULATION OF ADAPTIVE BEHAVIOUR – SAB'06.

[43] Muthuswamy, B. Implementing central pattern generators for bipedal walkers using cellular neural networks. Masters thesis. Berkeley, CA-USA: University of California, Department of Electrical Engineering and Computer Sciences; 2005.

[44] Billard, A. & Ijspeert, A. (2000). Biologically inspired neural controllers for motor control in a quadruped robot. Proceedings of the International Joint Conference on Neural Network IJCNN'2000, Come-Italy.

[45] Marder, E., Bucher, D., Schulz, D. & Taylor, A. (2005). Invertebrate central pattern generation moves along. *Current Biology, Vol. 15*, pp. 685-699.

[46] Cappelletto, J. Generator of gait modes for a quadruped robot based on neuro-physiological principles. Masters thesis. Caracas-Venezuela: Simón Bolívar University, Department of Electronics Engineering; 2007.

[47] Righetti, L. & Ijspeert, A. (2006). Programmable central pattern generators: an application to biped locomotion control. Proceedings of the IEEE International Conference on Robotics and Automation ICRA'2006, Orlando, FL-USA, pp. 1585-1590.

[48] ISO 10328: Prosthetics – Structural testing of lower limb prostheses – Requirements and test methods; 2006.

[49] Radcliffe, C. W. (1994). Four-bar linkage prosthetic knee mechanisms: kinematics, alignment and prescription criteria. *Prosthetics and Orthotics, Vol. 18*, 159-173.

[50] Genium (2015): Bionic Prosthetic System. Genium – Otto Bock [online]. Available from: http://genium.ottobock.com/en/the-genium/ (accessed January 30, 2015).

[51] Rheo Knee (2015): Bionic Technology. Rheo knee – Ossur [online]. Available from: http://www.ossur.com/prosthetic-solutions/bionic-technology/rheo-knee (accessed January 30, 2015).

[52] Power Knee (2015): Bionic Technology. Power knee – Ossur [online]. Available from: http://www.ossur.com/prosthetic-solutions/bionic-technology/power-knee (accessed January 30, 2015).

[53] Sup, F., Varol, H. A., Mitchell, J., Withrow, T. J. & Goldfarb, M. (2009). Preliminary evaluations of a self-contained anthropomorphic transfemoral prosthesis. *IEEE/ASME Transactions on Mechatronics, Vol. 14, No. 6*, pp. 667–676.

[54] Luinge, H. Inertial sensing of human movement. Doctoral thesis. Twente-The Netherlands: University of Twente; 2002.

[55] Roetenberg, D. Inertial and magnetic sensing of human motion. Doctoral thesis. Twente-The Netherlands: University of Twente; 2006.

[56] Torrealba, R. R., Castellano, J. M., Fernández-López, G. & Grieco, J. C. (2007). Characterisation of gait cycle from accelerometer data. *Electronics Letter, Vol. 43, No. 20*, pp. 1066-1068.

[57] Torrealba, R. R., Cappelletto, J., Fermín, L., Grieco, J. C. & Fernández-López, G. (2010). Statistics-based technique for automated detection of gait events from accelerometer signals. *Electronics Letters, Vol. 46, No. 22*, pp. 1483-1485.

[58] Torrealba, R. R., Cappelletto, J., González, A. & Fermín-León, L. (2010). Detecting human gait cycle sub-phases from lower limb acceleration signals using k-means algorithm. Proceedings of the International Conference on Applied Bionics and Biomechanics ICABB'2010, Venice-Italy, pp. 1-8.

[59] Endolite (2015): Orion2 [online]. Available from: http://www.endolite.com/products /orion2 (accessed January 23, 2015).

[60] Nordin, M. & Frankel, V. H. Basic biomechanics of the musculoskeletal system. Philadelphia, PA-USA: Lippincott Williams & Wilkins; 2001.

[61] Bar, A., Ishai, G., Meretsky, P. & Koren, Y. (1983). Adaptive microcomputer control of an artificial knee in level walking. *Journal of Biomedical Engineering (now called Medical Engineering & Physics), No. 5*, pp. 145-150.

[62] Aeyels, B., Peeraer, L., Sloten, J. & Van der Perre, G. (1992). Development of an above-knee prosthesis equipped with a microcomputer-controlled knee joint: first test results. *Journal of Biomedical Engineering, No. 14*, pp. 199-202.

[63] Jeong-Jung, K. & Ju-Jang, L. (2007). Gait adaptation method of biped robot for various terrains using central pattern generator (CPG) and learning mechanism. Proceedings of the International Conference on Control, Automation and Systems ICCAS'07, Seoul-Korea, pp. 10-14.

[64] Kimura, H., Fukuoka, Y., Hada, Y. & Takase, K. (2002). Three-dimensional adaptive dynamic walking of a quadruped - rolling motion feedback to cpgs controlling pitching

motion. Proceedings of the IEEE International Conference on Robotics and Automation ICRA'2002, Washington, DC-USA, pp. 2228-2233.

[65] Cappelletto, J., Estévez, P., Medina, W., Fermín, L., Bogado, J. M., Grieco, J. C. & Fernández-López, G. (2006). Gait synthesis and modulation for quadruped robot locomotion using a simple feed-forward network. Proceedings of the 8th International Conference on Artificial Intelligence and Soft Computing ICAISC'2006, Zakopane-Poland, pp. 731-739.

[66] Chiel, H., Beer, R. & Gallagher, J. (1999). Evolution and analysis of model CPGs for walking I: dynamical modules. *Journal of Computational Neuroscience, Vol. 7, No. 2*, pp. 99-118.

[67] Nakanishi, J., Morimoto, J., Endo, G., Cheng, G., Schaal, S. & Kawato, M. (2004). An empirical exploration of phase resetting for robust biped locomotion with dynamical movement primitives. Proceedings of the IEEE/RSJ International Conference on Intelligent Robots and Systems IROS'2004, Sendai-Japan, pp. 919-924.

[68] Cappelletto, J., Estévez, P., Fernández-López, G. & Grieco, J. C. (2007). A CPG with force feedback for a statically stable quadruped gait. Proceedings of the 10th International Conference on Climbing and Walking Robots and the Supporting Technologies for Mobile Machines CLAWAR'2007, Singapore-Singapore, pp. 37-46.

[69] Torrealba, R. R., Cappelletto, J., Fermín, L., Fernández-López, G. & Grieco, J. C. (2012). Cybernetic knee prosthesis: application of an adaptive central pattern generator. *Kybernetes: The International Journal of Systems & Cybernetics, Vol. 41, No. 1/2*, pp. 192-205.

[70] Nakanishi, J., Morimoto, J., Endo, G., Cheng, G., Schaal, S. & Kawato, M. (2004). Learning from demonstration and adaptation of biped locomotion. *Robotics and Autonomous Systems, Vol. 47*, pp. 79-91.

[71] Korioth, T. W. & Versluis, A. (1997). Modeling the mechanical behavior of the jaws and their related structures by finite element (Fe) analysis. *Critical reviews in oral biology & medicine, Vol. 8, No. 1*, pp. 90-104.

[72] Ha, S. K., Keilers, C. & Chang, F. (1992). Finite element analysis of composite structures containing distributed piezoceramic sensors and actuators. *AIAA Journal, Vol. 30, No. 3*, pp. 772-780.

[73] Torrealba, R. R., Zambrano, L. A. & Messingher, G. (2012). Optimización del chasis de una exoprótesis de rodilla utilizando la interacción directa entre programas de diseño en 3D y análisis de esfuerzos por MEF (Optimization of chassis of a knee exoprosthesis using direct interaction between softwares of 3D design and stress analysis by FEM). Proceedings of the XI Congreso Internacional de Métodos Numéricos en Ingeniería y Ciencias Aplicadas CIMENICS'2012, Porlamar-Venezuela, pp. BSB 1-6.

[74] Wolf, S., Eiberger, O. & Hirzinger, G. (2011). The DLR FSJ: energy based design of a variable stiffness joint. Proceedings of the IEEE International Conference on Robotics and Automation ICRA'2011, Shanghai-China, pp. 5082-5089.

[75] Vanderborght, B., Albu-Schäffer, A., Bicchi, A., Burdet, E., Caldwell, D. G., Carloni, R., Catalano, M., Eiberger, O., Friedl, W., Ganesh, G., Garabini, M., Grebenstein, M., Grioli, G., Haddadin, S., Hoppner, H., Jafari, A., Laffranchi, M., Lefeber, D., Petit, F., Stramigioli, S., Tsagarakis, N., Van Damme, M., Van Ham, R., Visser, L. C. & Wolf, S. (2013). Variable impedance actuators: A review. *Robotics and Autonomous Systems,*

ISSN 09218890 [online]. Available from: http://linkinghub.elsevier.com/retrieve/pii/S0921889013001188.

[76] Tagliamonte, N. L., Sergi, F., Accoto, D., Carpino, G. & Guglielmelli, E. (2012). Double actuation architectures for rendering variable impedance in compliant robots: A review. *Mechatronics, Vol. 22, No. 8*, pp. 1187-1203. ISSN 09574158 [online]. Available from: http://linkinghub.elsevier.com/retrieve/pii/S0957415812001493.

[77] Petit, F., Chalon, M., Friedl, W., Grebenstein, M., Albu-Schäffer, A. & Hirzinger, G. (2010). Bidirectional antagonistic variable stiffness actuation: analysis, design & implementation. Proceedings of the IEEE International Conference on Robotics and Automation ICRA'2010, Anchorage, AK-USA, pp. 4189-4196.

[78] Friedl, W., Höppner, H., Petit, F. & Hirzinger, G. (2011). Wrist and forearm rotation of the DLR hand arm system: mechanical design, shape analysis and experimental validation. Proceedings of the IEEE/RSJ International Conference on Intelligent Robots and Systems IROS'2011, San Francisco, CA-USA, pp. 1836-1842.

[79] Petit, F., Friedl, W., Höppner, H. & Grebenstein, M. (2015). Analysis and synthesis of the bidirectional antagonistic variable stiffness mechanism. *IEEE/ASME Transactions on Mechatronics, Vol. 20, No. 2*, pp. 684-695.

[80] Torrealba, R. R. & Udelman, S. B. (2015). Design of cam shape for maximum stiffness variability on a novel compliant actuator using differential evolution. *Mechanism and machine theory* (in review).

In: New Developments in Knee Prosthesis Research
Editor: Janice Stewart
ISBN: 978-1-63482-700-3

Chapter 2

Development of Mechanical Polycentric Knee Prosthesis: Introducing a Methodological Approach

Belkys T. Amador[1,2]***, Rafael R. Torrealba***[1]
and Carmen M. Müller-Karger[1]
[1]Biomechanics Research Group,
Simón Bolívar University, Caracas, Venezuela
[2]Prototypes Laboratory,
National Experimental University of Táchira, San Cristóbal, Venezuela

Abstract

According to a survey done in the literature on the field until 2010, design of 4-bar mechanisms for polycentric knee prostheses was performed heuristically. Therefore, the main motivation of this work was to determine aspects of the design process on this kind of prosthetic devices suitable of a technical approach, which could go far beyond from a simple empirical point of view. Knee prostheses must comply several basic characteristics in order to provide a safe and biomechanical performance to its user during walking, these are: 1. stability during load response, 2. easy flexion during late stance and pre-swing, 3. recover of extension during late swing before next contact, and 4. proper resistance to critical loading. From these, 1 and 2 might be related to the location of the instantaneous center of rotation (ICR) of the prosthesis with regard to the ground reaction force (GRF) line during the stance phase of gait cycle [1]. The third aspect requires the proper analysis of forces and moments of the assistant extension mechanism (AEM) respect to the ICR and the latter requires a detailed structural stress analysis of the device. For proper kinematical functioning, dimensions of the 4 linkages of the mechanism must be set, as well as the angular position of the prosthesis on the leg. This renders a multi-dimensional search problem that is complex to solve. Nonetheless, artificial intelligence techniques have emerged as a very good alternative to carry out this kind of searches. In particular, genetic algorithms (GAs) perform a search with bias in a multi-dimensional space of solutions. In this work, the aforementioned dimensions of the mechanism, targeting a specific trajectory of the ICR, were gauged by a particularly programmed GA integrated with gait analysis data on a computing platform. Later, a structural analysis of the prosthesis was performed via finite element method [2,3], according to the requirements of the standard ISO 10328 [4]. And finally, a functional prototype was manufactured and adapted to two unilateral transfemoral amputees, which allowed assessing the performance of the design qualitatively, using questionnaire, and quantitatively, via gait analysis. This work is based on a series of articles published by the co-authors on this matter, but at the same time, it is a new text never published before as a whole, as this presents all the content brought out by this project up-to-now for the first time.

1. Introduction

The main objective of a prosthetic application after lower limb amputation is to enable the patient to stand, to walk again as close as possible to a normal human gait and finally, to restore the cosmetics through the recovery of body symmetry. Within the lower limb prosthesis, the knee joint is the one that has the function of providing stability in stance phase and controlling the swing phase during walking [5]; these functions can be performed by mechanical or smart devices. Prosthetic knees are classified according to the number of axes as monocentric or polycentric [6]. For a monocentric one, flexion and extension occur around a single axis. For a polycentric one, the axis of the joint moves depending on the angle of knee flexion, i.e., there is an instantaneous center of rotation [1].

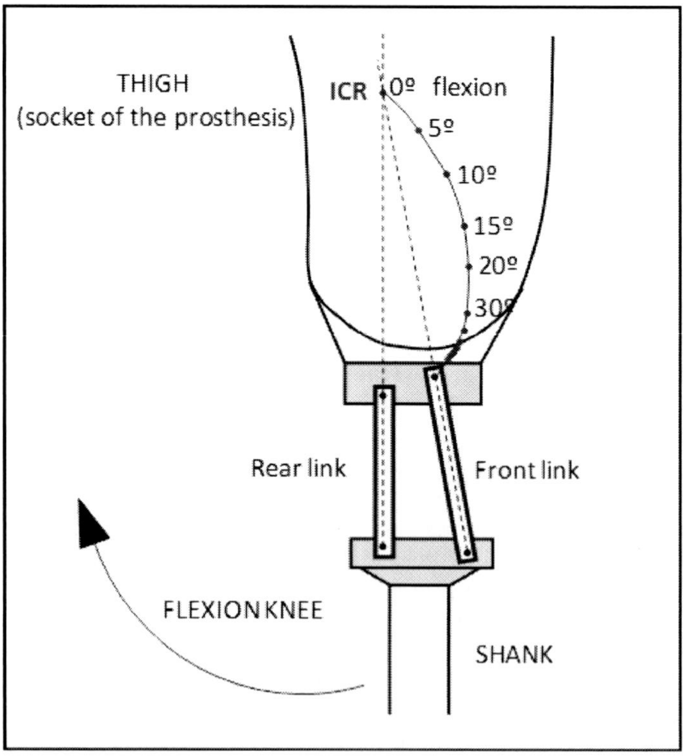

Figure 1. Range of motion of the ICR on a polycentric knee prosthesis (adapted from [7]).

This axis is located, for any angle of knee flexion, at the intersection of the extensions of the centerlines of front and rear links of the mechanism, such as shown in Figure 1. More in detail, in the same figure it can be noticed that as the knee flexion angle increases, the ICR draws a forward and downward trajectory.

In general, comparing pure mechanical mechanisms, the following advantages for a polycentric knee mechanism (PKM) in relation to one with a single center might be listed [8,9]:

- PKM increases stability at heel strike, due to the possibility of placing the ICR posterior to the load line of the mechanism. For the monocentric prosthesis, the rotation center has a fixed position and to ensure stability, amputee needs to apply a considerable hip extension moment.
- PKM shortens the length of the prosthesis during the swing phase, ensuring proper foot-ground distance to prevent stumbling. Research by [7] showed that 4-bars knees provide larger foot-floor distance, from 0.9 to 3.2 cm more than the corresponding monocentric prostheses.
- PKM improves cosmetics during flexion, especially important in the sitting position (90° flexion), as the mechanism allows the leg to locate behind the thigh.
- PKM presents a more natural behavior that monocentric during flexion, as this performs movements of rotation and translation simultaneously.

The development of external knee prostheses using polycentric mechanisms has been addressed in the works of [10-16], however, none of these makes a reference to fundamental aspects of prostheses design nor to mechanisms sizing, including its kinematics and stability analysis. Radcliffe [1] emphasizes that small differences in the length of the links of a PKM as well as the position of the joints between them, may result in large changes in the kinematics of the mechanism and thus directly affect its stability. Hence, through the configuration and sizing of a PKM, the location of ICR in each phase of gait can be manipulated, allowing voluntary control of the prosthesis by the amputee, avoiding, for example, that for some flexion angles the knee buckles, as the ICR meets the load line in an inappropriate manner. In Gonzalez Lugo's work [17], for instance, the design of 4-bar mechanisms for prosthetic knees is addressed using genetic algorithms, nonetheless, the considerations are for a general application mechanism and the sizing is not suited for a knee prosthesis [18].

Radcliffe [1] suggests that the direction of the GRF line viewed in the sagittal plane is directly related to the stability offered by a knee during walking and that the orientation of the load line may be controlled by the amputee by applying hip flexion or extension moments. In the PKM, after heel strike and during load response, the ICR should be located posterior to the load line to ensure stability of the knee. Subsequently, its location must be prior to the load line, to initiate voluntary flexion during terminal stance and pre-swing, before takeoff. Therefore, controlling the ICR in relation to the GRF position allows the manipulation of hip moment magnitude the amputee must exert to control the stability of the prosthesis as well as subsequent flexion. Figure 2 shows the stability analysis on a PKM.

From this information and knowing that during prosthesis design the dimensioning to guarantee proper kinematic behavior (kinematic sizing) is traditionally empiric and/or based on the size and configuration of commercially available prostheses [10-16], a rigorous methodology for kinematic sizing of a 4-bar mechanism is presented in this chapter and applied during the design of a polycentric knee prosthesis. The goal of this research was to comprehensively size such PKM with six parameters that define its configuration, for which it was developed a computing platform featured by: (1) application of principles of the mechanism stability during stance phase of gait cycle, (2) use of gait analysis data as input from a transfemoral amputee and (3) introduction of an artificial intelligence technique.

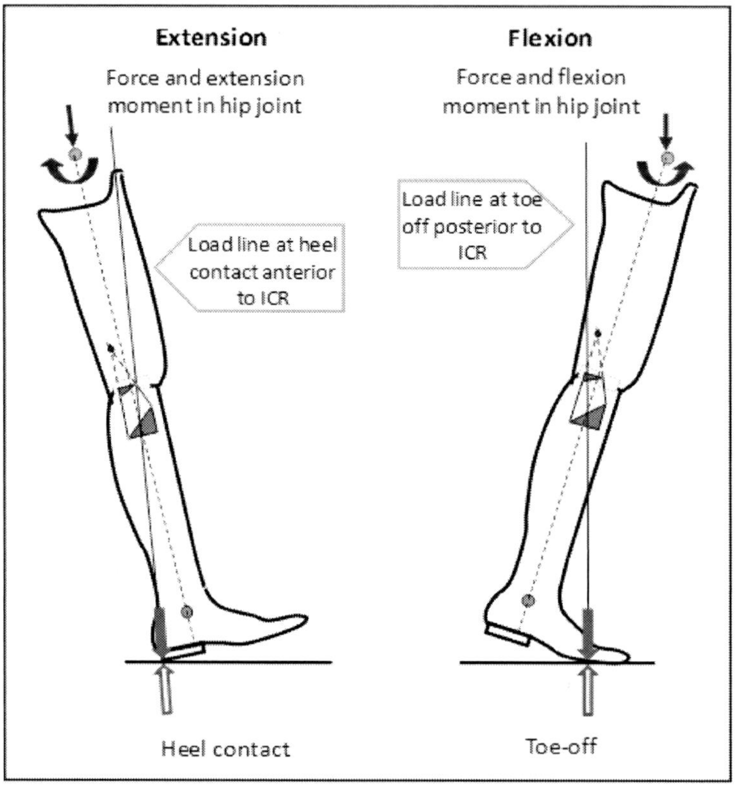

Figure 2. Stability analysis of a PKM with voluntary control (adapted from [1]).

2. Methodology

The development of the polycentric knee began with the conceptual design, for which the needs of transfemoral amputees were identified and the goals were outlined through the design specifications. Then, the detailed design process of the prosthesis was performed in three steps, first by determining the proper dimensions to fulfill the kinematical needs of the mechanism; second, by sizing the device under a structural point of view; and lastly, by designing an AEM. Parts of the prosthesis and the AEM were manufactured, subsequently an assembled prototype was adjusted, and finally the prosthesis was tested, initially using a prosthesis simulator and later by unilateral transfemoral amputees. Figure 3 shows the described process.

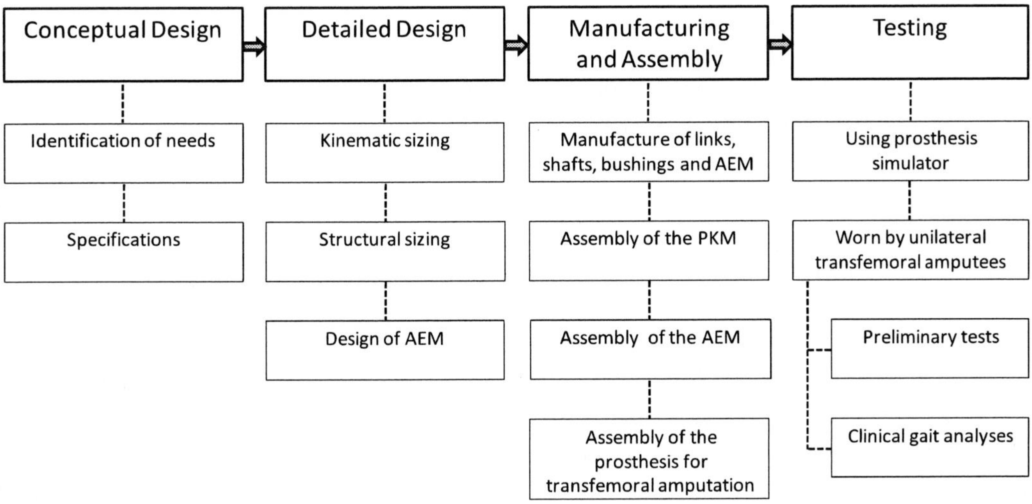

Figure 3. Methodological process for the development of the polycentric knee prosthesis.

2.1. Conceptual Design

A survey done to a group of transfemoral amputated patients in Venezuela led to identify needs and specifications for the conceptual design of the prosthetic knee [19]. All patients were experienced lower limb prosthesis users for more than six months, and aged between 18 and 70 years. As a result, the variables on which patients placed greater emphasis were prostheses security during stance; functionality, emphasizing that it should resemble the behavior of a healthy joint, i.e., offer flexion control and security in stance phase as well as having assistance to the extent in swing phase; and finally, personal monetary investment required to get access to the device. On this basis, a polycentric 4-bar mechanism that provides voluntary control to users was pursued in this project. Design specifications were stablished as follows:

Mandatory:

- Behavior of the prosthesis mechanism must be polycentric and resemble the one of a sound knee as much as possible.
- Mobility grade of the prosthesis must correspond to Grade 2 in the *Medicare Functional Classification Level* (MFCL) scale.
- Maximum knee flexion angle must be at least 110°.
- Prosthesis must support loads applied by a person weighing 100 kg during walking.

Wants:

- Materials required to produce the prosthesis are resistant to corrosion and oxidation, easy-to-machine and found in domestic market.
- Manufacturing processes employed are conventional, as metal-machining and bolted joints.

Nice-to-haves:

- Knee prosthesis weighs no more than 1 kg.
- Prosthesis presents standard dimensions of commercial adaptors to ease its connection with other prosthetic components.

2.2. Details Design

2.2.1. Kinematic Sizing of the Mechanism

To size the mechanism for a proper kinematic behavior a mathematical model was programmed in a computing platform, using MATLAB® version R2009b. As shown in Figure 4, an iterative process includes the application of a GA that proposes dimensions for the six parameters required to defining the mechanism. This set of parameters, as well as the equations governing kinematics of the 4-bar mechanism and the kinematic and kinetic data generated from gait analysis of a patient with unilateral transfemoral amputation, are fed into the computing platform. With such information, the platform reproduces the actual movement of the leg during the stance phase in the sagittal plane, as well as the position of the GRF and the configuration of the prosthesis mechanism on the leg with respect to the ICR, allowing a visual comparison of the latter relative to the GRF.

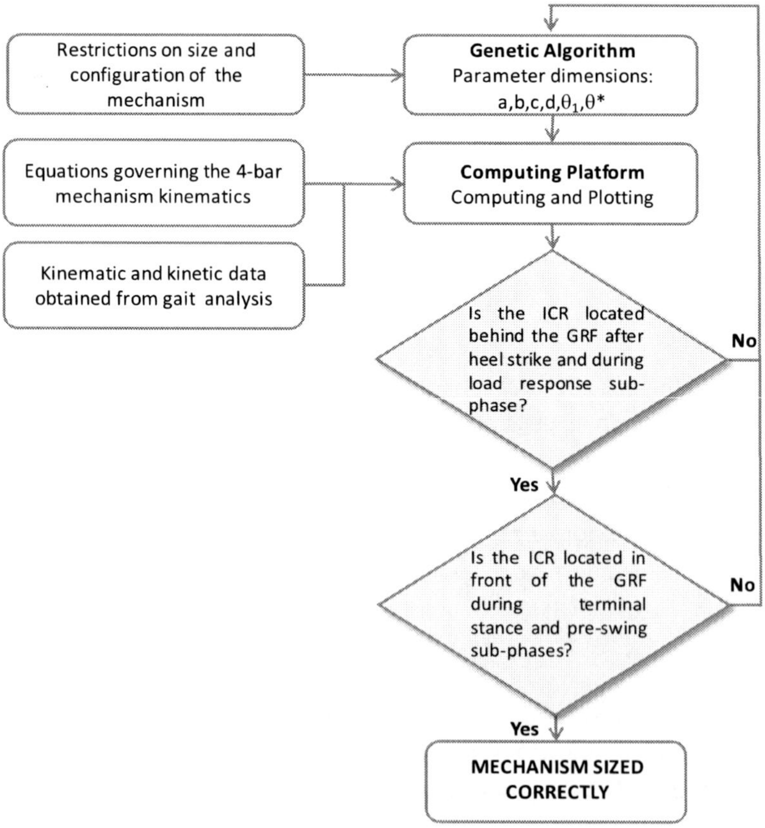

Figure 4. Methodological process for kinematic sizing of the mechanism.

The stability of the PKM is guaranteed when the ICR is located behind the GRF after heel strike and during load response sub-phase [1]. Similarly, if the ICR is located in front of the GRF during terminal stance and pre-swing sub-phases, the mechanism allows voluntary flexion before toe-off to start swing phase of gait cycle. If the computed design solution complies these two conditions, the mechanism is deemed correctly sized; otherwise, the sizing is discarded and a new set of six parameters is requested to the GA and the iteration process begins again. Actually, regarding the functionality of the GA, deeper insight will be given in the following lines as it is more complex than what has been just said.

2.2.1.1. Gait Analysis as Input to the Computing Platform

Clinical gait analysis was performed on an unilateral transfemoral amputee after signing the corresponding informed consent. By the moment of the testing, the patient had three years of experience using commercial 4-bars polycentric prosthetic knees. Helen Hayes protocol for full-body biomechanical model using reflective markers spread across different points of interest was applied [20]. Kinematics data throughout the gait cycle was obtained from both lower limbs. And data was processed using the CORTEX® software provided by MotionAnalysis Corp. Figure 5 presents one of the collected gait cycles showing the GRF from the force plates and the full-body joints. The graphs at the bottom of the screen represent the kinematic motion of the prosthetic knee.

Combining anterior-posterior and vertical components of the GRF vector with the center of pressure in the sagittal plane, the graphical representation of the spatio-temporal sequence of GRF during the stance phase of gait cycle was obtained. This representation (Figure 6a) is known as Butterfly diagram or Pedotti diagram [21]. On the other hand, using hip, knee and ankle center coordinates in the sagittal plane, actual movement of the lower limb during the stance phase of gait cycle is plotted in Figure 6b. This couple of figures is superimposed later, together with the mechanism of the prosthesis, with the aim at evaluating the behavior of the designed mechanism.

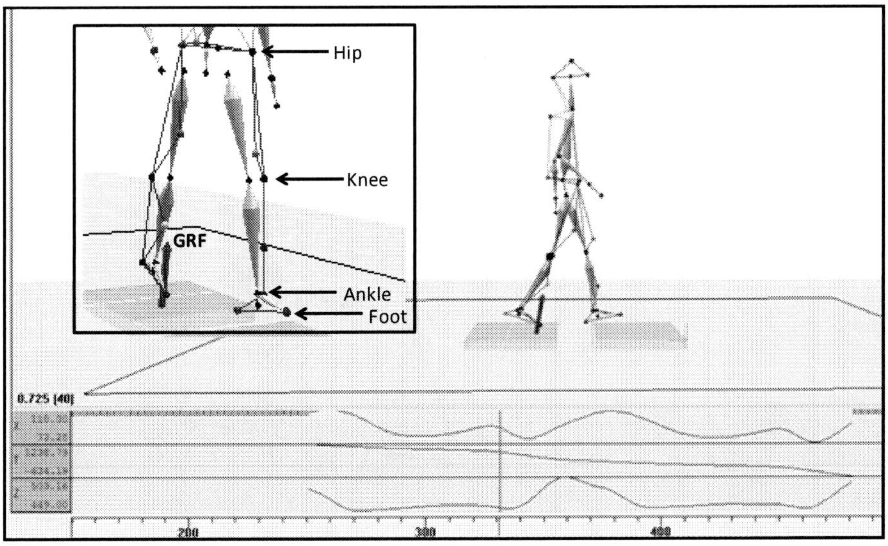

Figure 5. One of the collected gait cycles from clinical gait analysis on an unilateral transfemoral amputee.

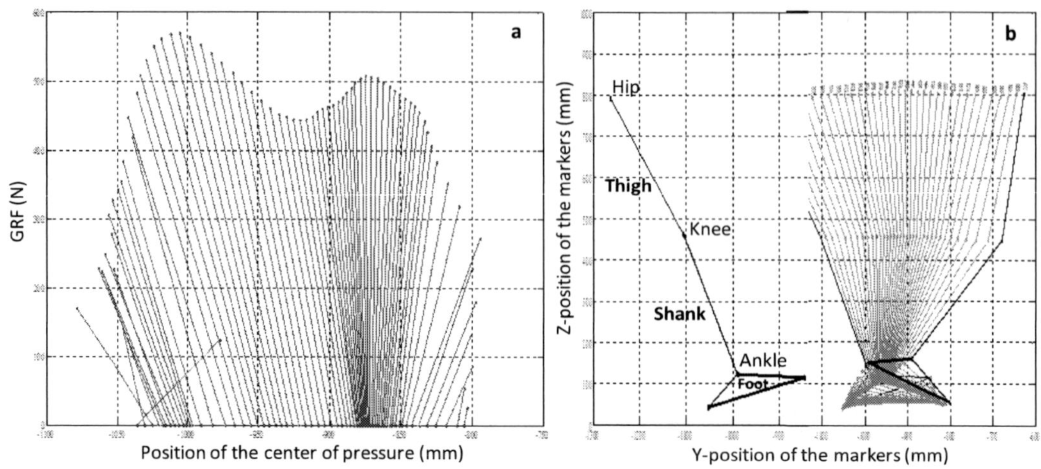

Figure 6. (a) Representation of the spatio-temporal sequence of GRF along gait cycle, (b) Movement of the lower limb during the stance phase of gait cycle.

2.2.1.2. Governing Equations

To represent the mechanism and its ICR, a general mechanism configuration shown in Figure 7 was used, the four links are hinged together as follows : 'a' to 'b' by pin A, 'b' with 'c' by pin B, 'c' with 'd' by pin O_B and 'd' with 'a' by pin O_A. Following the methodology designated by [22], the link 'd' is considered to be attached to the lower leg (extensor tube of the prosthesis to the foot) and fixed to the ground in order to analyze the mechanism stability, while the link 'b' is attached to the thigh (socket of the prosthesis) and considered as the moving link yielding the knee flexion angle.

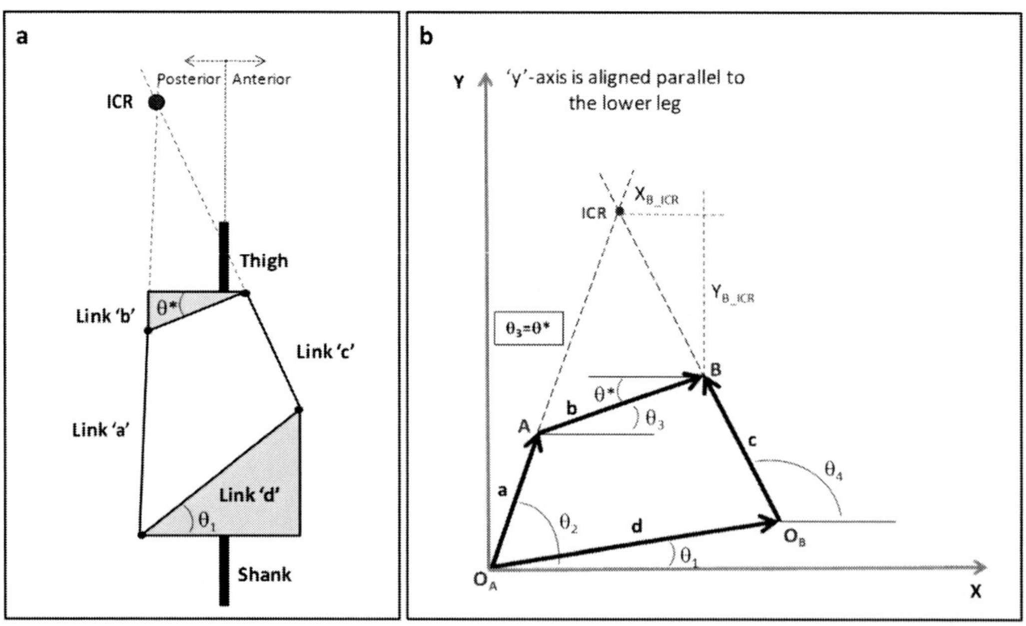

Figure 7. (a) General configuration of the mechanism, (b) Geometric representation of the mechanism.

The variable θ^* is an angle to design the link 'b' and is measured with origin at pin B, the variable θ_1 is the design angle for link 'd' which is measured with origin at pin O_A, the ICR is located at the intersection of the extensions of links 'a' and 'c' . The angle θ_3 is an independent variable because it is associated with link 'b' (fixed to the thigh) and represent the input motion to the mechanism. The mathematical equations proposed by [23] to determine configuration and kinematics of a 4-bar mechanism are used to calculate the unknown variables θ_2 and θ_4 (equations 1 and 5 respectively) when the lengths of the four links 'a', 'b', 'c' and 'd', the input angle θ_3 and the design angles θ_1 and θ^* are known. The variables θ_2 and θ_4 are the angles between links 'a' and 'c' with the horizontal reference line respectively, both measured counter-clockwise as shown in Figure 7b. The origin of the coordinate system is located in the lower-back corner at pin O_A (see Figure 7b).

$$\theta_2 = 2\,tan^{-1}\left[\frac{-B \pm \sqrt{B^2 - 4AC}}{2A}\right] \quad (1)$$

with:

$$A = (a^2 + b^2 - c^2 + d^2)/(2ab) - d(cos\,\theta_1\,cos\,\theta_3 + sin\,\theta_1\,sin\,\theta_3)/a - cos\,\theta_3 + d\,cos\,\theta_1/b \quad (2)$$

$$B = 2\,(sin\,\theta_3 - d\,sin\,\theta_1/b) \quad (3)$$

$$C = (a^2 + b^2 - c^2 + d^2)/(2ab) - d(cos\,\theta_1\,cos\,\theta_3 + sin\,\theta_1\,sin\,\theta_3)/a + cos\,\theta_3 - d\,cos\,\theta_1/b \quad (4)$$

$$\theta_4 = 2\,tan^{-1}\left[\frac{-E \pm \sqrt{E^2 - 4DF}}{2D}\right] \quad (5)$$

with:

$$D = (b^2 - a^2 + c^2 + d^2)/(2bc) - d(cos\,\theta_1\,cos\,\theta_3 + sin\,\theta_1\,sin\,\theta_3)/c - d\,cos\,\theta_1/b + cos\,\theta_3 \quad (6)$$

$$E = 2\,(d\,sin\,\theta_1/b - sin\,\theta_3) \quad (7)$$

$$F = (b^2 - a^2 + c^2 + d^2)/(2bc) - d(cos\,\theta_1\,cos\,\theta_3 + sin\,\theta_1\,sin\,\theta_3)/c + d\,cos\,\theta_1/b - cos\,\theta_3 \quad (8)$$

Input angle θ_3 is equal to the sum of the flexion angle θ_R and the design angle θ^*. The knee flexion angle is obtained from the gait analysis described previously. Given the equations 9, 10, 11 and 12, the calculated angles θ_2 and θ_4 are then used to calculate the vertex coordinates of the mechanism (X_{OA}, Y_{OA}), (X_{OB}, Y_{OB}), (X_A , Y_A) and (X_B, Y_B), for its graphical representation.

$$X_{O_A} = 0; \; Y_{O_A} = 0 \quad (9)$$

$$X_{O_B} = d\cos\theta_1\,;\; Y_{O_B} = d\sin\theta_1 \tag{10}$$

$$X_A = a\cos\theta_2;\; Y_A = a\sin\theta_2 \tag{11}$$

$$X_B = X_{O_B} + c\cos\theta_4;\; Y_B = Y_{O_B} + c\sin\theta_4 \tag{12}$$

The reference coordinates system of the mechanism was fixed to the lower segment of the prosthetic moving leg (see Figure 8). Pin B, belonging to the link 'b', is considered the anatomic center of the knee (this point is the mechanism reference for prosthetic knee alignment [7,24]. Reference 'y'-axis is aligned parallel to the lower leg and 'x'-axis is perpendicular to the former and pointing forward.

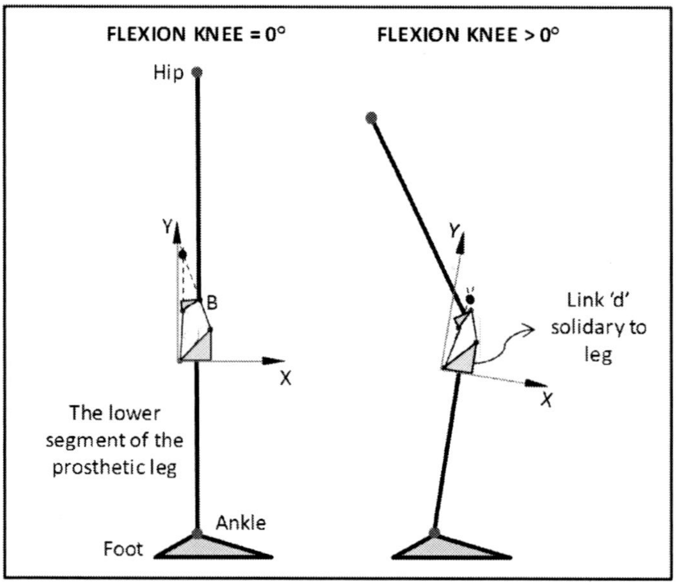

Figure 8. Schematic representation of the mechanism placed on the leg.

More in detail, to define the mechanism dimensions efficiently, and overcome the problem complexity of working simultaneously with 6 parameters: lengths of the four links 'a', 'b', 'c' and 'd' and the angles θ_1 and θ^*, a GA was used as follows. First, to set a reference, the position of ICR for each knee flexion angle is measured respect to pin B; calculated horizontally by equation 13 (X_{B_ICR}) and vertically by equation 14 (Y_{B_ICR}), as shown in Figure 5.

$$X_{B\_ICR} = \frac{(X_{O_B}\tan\theta_4 - Y_{O_B})}{(\tan\theta_4 - \tan\theta_2)} - d\cos\theta_1 - c\cos\theta_4 \tag{13}$$

$$Y_{B\_ICR} = \frac{(X_{OB}\tan\theta_4 - Y_{OB})\tan\theta_2}{(\tan\theta_4 - \tan\theta_2)} - d\sin\theta_1 - c\sin\theta_4 \tag{14}$$

Also, the following additional constraints were included:

1. For a voluntary control mechanism [1], the length of the posterior link (link ‘a’) must be greater than the front link length (link ‘c’).
2. To ensure continuous movement of the mechanism, the sum of the lengths of the shortest and longest links must be less than the sum of the lengths of the other two links (Grashof linkage condition [23]).
3. Minimum and maximum acceptable values were established for each of the 6 parameters of the mechanism as shown in Table 1. This definition was made considering physical dimensions of human leg.

Table 1. Dimensional range for each parameter

Parameter	Minimum value	Maximun value
Link a	15 mm	90 mm
Link b	20 mm	45 mm
Link c	15 mm	90 mm
Link d	15 mm	60 mm
Angle θ_1	0°	40°
Angle θ^*	0°	40°

2.2.1.3. Optimal Location of ICR

According to [1], smooth motion of ICR forward and downward as knee flexion angle increases is very important for voluntary control of a knee prosthesis. It is recommended that at heel contact with the leg in full extension, location of the ICR should be approximately 100 mm above the center of the knee (Y_{B_ICR}) and 6 mm posterior to the vertical reference line (X_{B_ICR}) . Moreover, Radcliffe points out as an appropriate location of ICR coordinates those of the *Hosmer Spectrum* prosthetic knee: with 128 mm for vertical position (Y_{B_ICR}) and 20 mm behind the vertical reference line (X_{B_ICR}) [24]; he also notes that, in order to increase the stability, ICR must have almost a constant height (distance in 'y') at least for the first 5° of knee flexion.

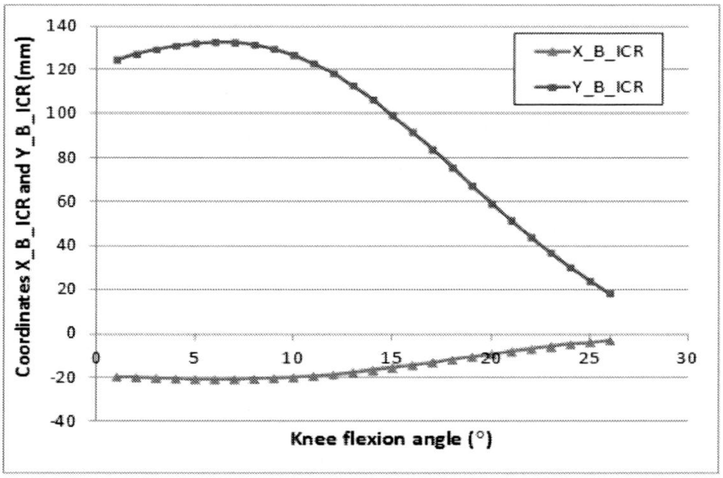

Figure 9. Reference curves for ICR location with respect to vertex B, X_{B_CIR} and Y_{B_CIR}, resulting from procedure shown in [25].

From this information, the ideal location for the ICR coordinates (X_{B_ICR} and Y_{B_ICR}) of the mechanism were set conveniently in relation to pin B for each knee flexion angle. Though further details about this particular procedure created by the co-authors is out of the scope of this chapter, should the reader need more information please refer to [25]. Figure 9 shows the ideal smooth curves of ICR location established. The X_{B_ICR} curve has little variation for the range of knee flexion, while Y_{B_ICR} to 0° of knee flexion starts approximately at 120 mm and tends to increase during the first 5° of flexion and then moves smoothly downward with successive flexion increment.

2.2.1.4. Programming the GA

The GA is employed as a random search technique for determining 6 design parameters of the mechanism simultaneously. For each synthesized GA solution, a resultant ICR curve is obtained, the subroutine evaluates quantitatively whether or not this solution get close to the desired ICR curves using an adaptive function or 'fitness'. This 'fitness' function is based on a metric approximation error curves, Y_{B_ICR} and X_{B_ICR}, therefore the GA becomes a multi-purpose technique for a minimization of the approximation error, where the different parameters must be constraint by the values described in Table 1, as well as the restrictions derived from the mechanism type -of voluntary control- and the Grashof linkage.

For the initial implementation of the GA, few generations where created with a small number of individuals and a low rate of mutation. However, considering the firsts results obtained change in the algorithm were necessary, including the contribution of different restrictions and increasing the number of generations and individuals to evaluate as many solutions as possible in a reasonable time, and also, to avoid falling into local minima variable mutation rate was implemented. The following details each of the main features of the algorithm:

1. Each chromosome (individual) is formed by 6 genes , one for each parameter 'a', 'b', 'c', 'd', θ1 and θ*; each gene had 2 bytes to ensure sufficient resolution for every parameter. The chromosome decoding was linear so all parameters were bounded between the values specified in Table 1.
2. The number of generations (iterations) was limited at 3,000, and each generation comprised 100 individuals (possible solutions).
3. As selecting technique, the 'Tournament' was used, i.e., all solutions have a non-zero probability of generating a seed for the next generation; even solutions with less fitness can provide advances when mixed with the rest of the population, leading to genetic variability of the population.
4. The mutation rate varies over time, for the first 10 generations 0.5 was used to obtain the most variable results and make a completely random search. From generation 11 the rate was lowered to 0.01 and every 100 generations the value of fitness of the best individual of the population was checked, for constant values of fitness the rate was increased in 0.005 until reach the generation 2,750. This was done to avoid the algorithm stay 'trapped' in a local minimum. Finally, from the 2,750 to the 3,000 generation, mutation rate was set at 0.0075.
5. Equation 15 is the generic fitness function used, the first 'fit_{xy}' relates to the calculation of the square mean error for X and Y considering the ICR curve obtained

by the GA and the ideal, using the equations 16 and 17. The error calculation is performed for each knee flexion angle θ_R. The other terms refer to the aforementioned restrictions applied on the runs to induce the GA to find the parameters of the mechanism that meet the desired performance. The term 'fit_{ac}' (constraint 1) refers to the restriction associated with voluntary control mechanism, where the rear link must be longer than the front one; the 'fit_{gr}' (constraint 2) relates to the Grashof linkage condition, where the sum of the lengths of the shortest and longest links must be less than the sum of the lengths of the other two links. Additionally the terms 'fit_{xicr}' (constraint 3) and 'fit_{yicr}' (constraint 4) were introduced to narrow the X_{B_ICR} and Y_{B_ICR} searching range within a tolerance band, respectively. Regarding the term 'fit_{an}' (constraint 5), it is introduced to restrict the width of the mechanism, whereas the term 'fit_{db}' (constraint 6) is introduced to force the link length 'd' to be greater than the length of link 'b'.

$$fit = \mathrm{fit_{xy}} + \mathrm{fit_{ac}} + \mathrm{fit_{gr}} + \mathrm{fit_{xicr}} + \mathrm{fit_{yicr}} + \mathrm{fit_{an}} + \mathrm{fit_{db}} \tag{15}$$

$$ex\_m = \sqrt{\frac{\sum_{i=0}^{\theta R}(x_{Di}-x_{Oi})^2}{N_{puntos}}} \tag{16}$$

$$ey\_m = \sqrt{\frac{\sum_{i=0}^{\theta R}(y_{Di}-y_{Oi})^2}{N_{puntos}}} \tag{17}$$

2.2.1.5. Results Obtained from the Use of GA and Computing Platform

The final solution was obtained after several iterations, adjustments to GA constraints and tuning of fitness equation while monitoring behavior of the ICR regarding the GRF on the computing platform, combined with resulting mechanism parameter dimensions suitable for manufacturing. Figure 10a represent the solution given by the GA subroutine (four links lengths and θ* and θ1 angles) considered as optimal and the resulting ICR location for knee flexion angle of 0°. Combining this configuration with the flexion angles θ_R obtained from the gait analysis, the successive movement of the mechanism from 0 to 90° of knee flexion is represented in Figure 10b (at intervals of 2°). Figure 11 shows the ICR trajectory for the final solution compared to the ideal described previously.

Figure 12 shows a graphical representation of the calculated mechanism placed on the leg (only frames 1, 5, 9 and 13 at 100 fps) and the GRF along the stance phase of gait cycle. It must be remarked that for the first 12 frames, approximately 10% of the gait cycle for the average walking speed of the patient of 0.91 m/s, the GRF vector is placed in front of the ICR, ensuring stability at initial contact and load response. A maximum knee flexion of 5° is achieved in these first 12 frames.

Then, in frame 55, approximately 45% of the gait cycle for the same walking speed, occurs maximum knee extension in the terminal stance (just before toe-off). From this frame, the GRF begins to get behind the ICR ensuring voluntary knee flexion, which is essential to initiate the swing phase. Figure 13 zooms in frames 1, 12 and 55; to detail the location of the ICR in relation to the GRF.

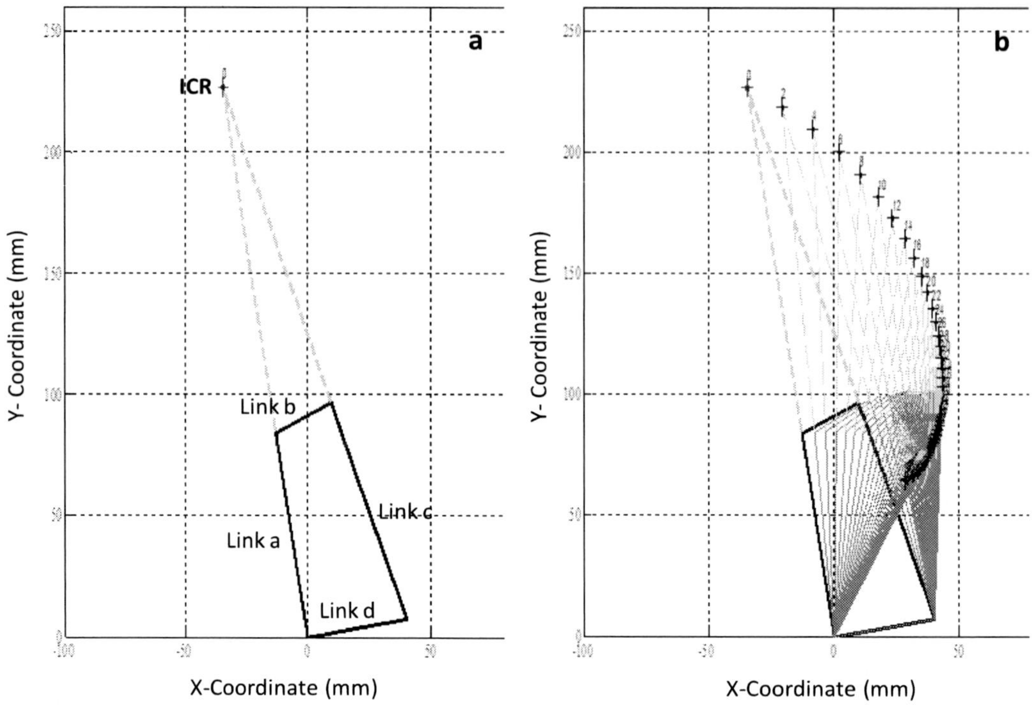

Figure 10. (a) Mechanism representation for 0° knee flexion, (b) Motion of the mechanism for knee flexion from 0 to 90°.

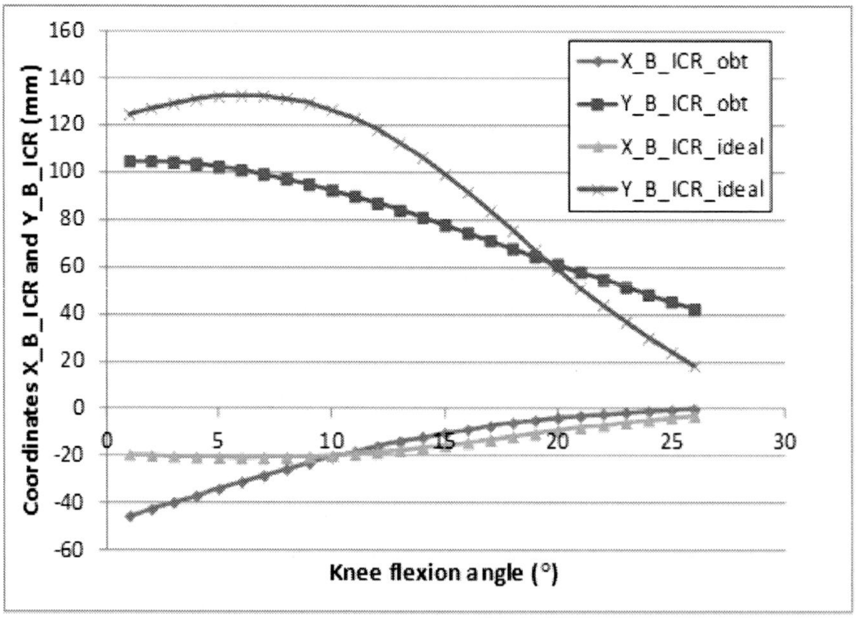

Figure 11. ICR coordinates for final solution compared to its desired position to ensure stability and voluntary control of the knee prosthesis.

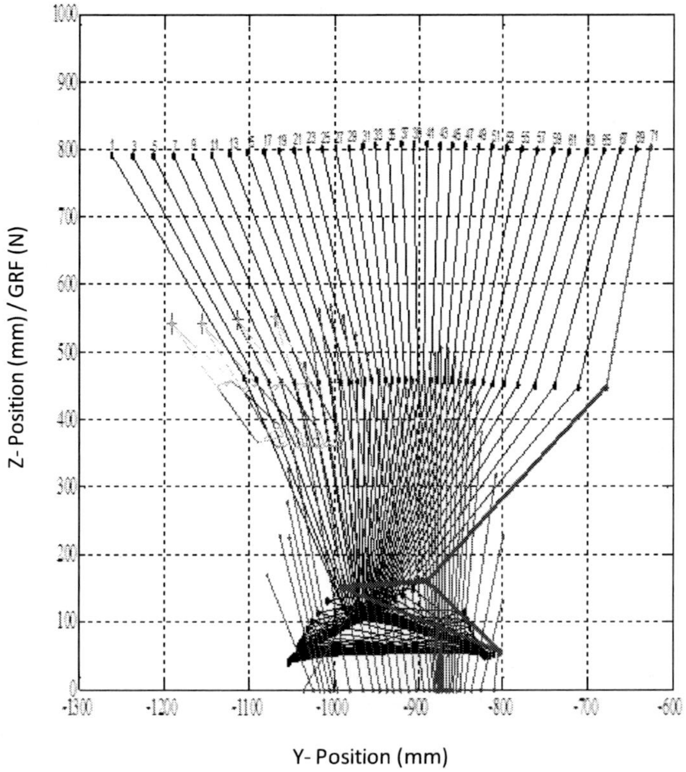

Figure 12. Graphical representation of the mechanism placed on the leg (for frames 1, 5, 9 and 13) and the location of the GRF along the stance phase of the gait cycle.

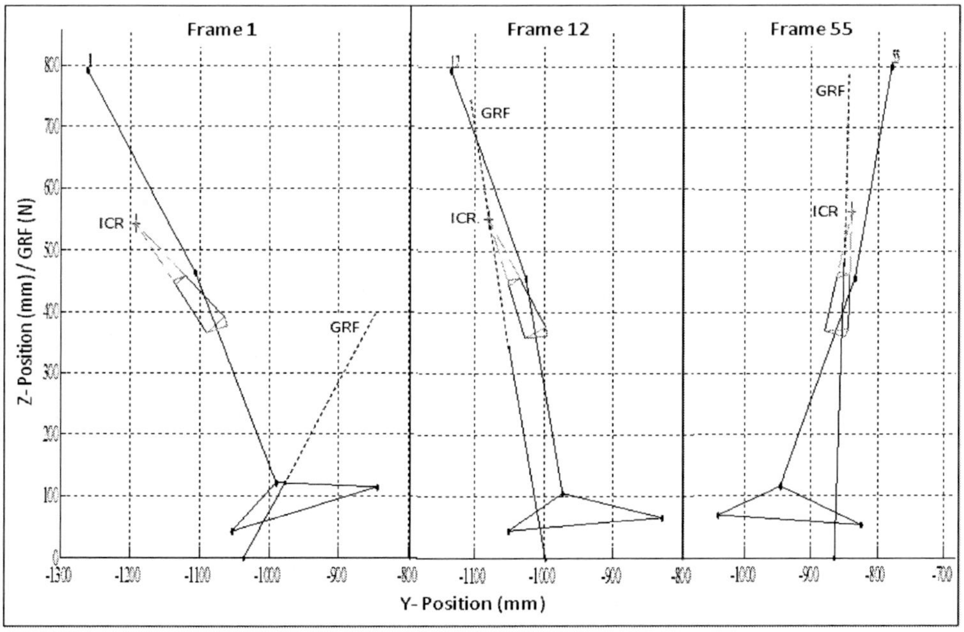

Figure 13. Representation of the mechanism of the prosthesis during the initial contact response (frame 1), loading response (frame 12) and in the final phase of support (frame 55).

2.2.2. Structural Sizing of the Mechanism

2.2.2.1. Preliminary Design of the Prototype

Considering the dimensions obtained for the 4-bar mechanism of the prosthesis, the physical dimensions of human leg and some references of commercial polycentric prostheses [26], a preliminary 3D CAD model of the prosthesis was developed as shown in Figure 14.

Two fundamental blocking surfaces were included within the design, the first one located behind link 'd' to limit full extension of the knee (equal to 0° flexion) and prevent hyperextension (see Figure 15a); the second one located behind link 'b' to limit maximum knee flexion set at 131.5° (see Figure 15b).

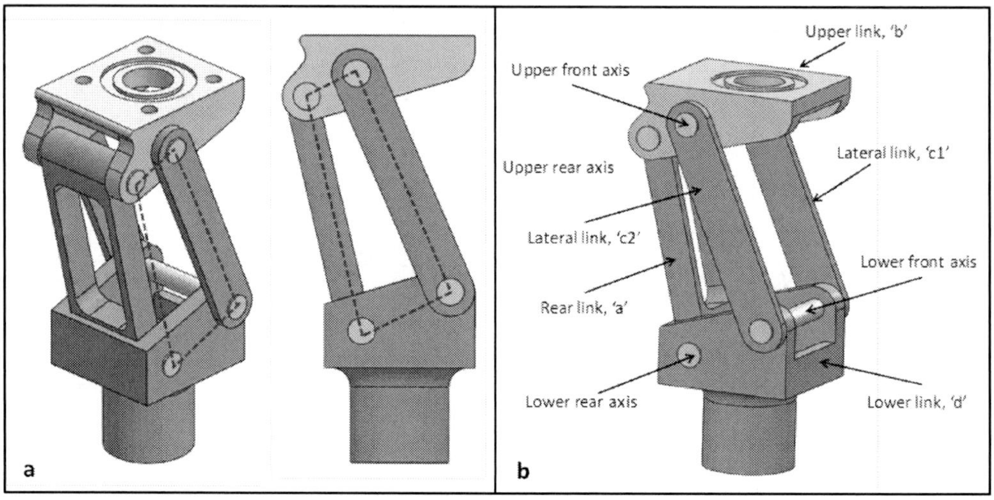

Figure 14. Preliminary 3D model of the knee prosthesis.

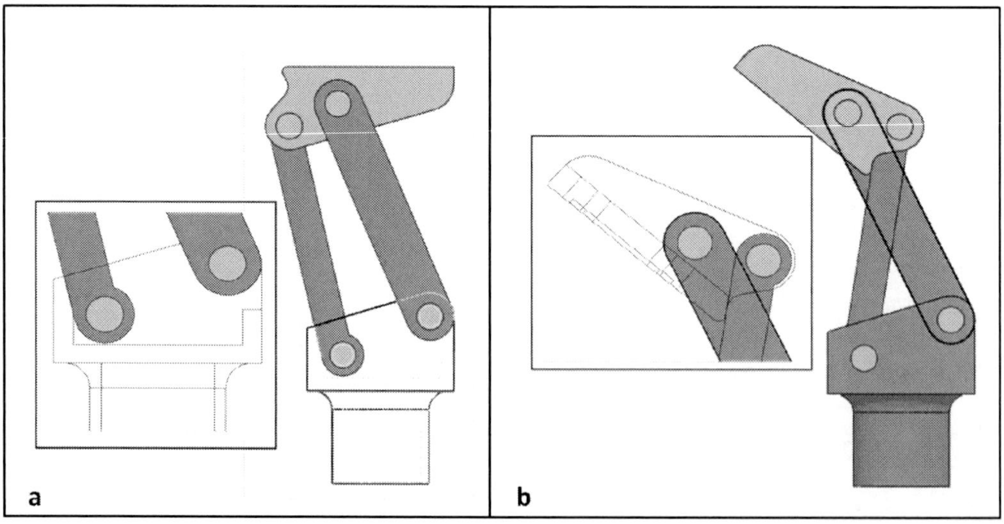

Figure 15. Blockade surfaces of the prosthesis: (a) Total knee extension, (b) Maximum flexion.

2.2.2.2. Stress Analyses of the Prostheses

Stress analysis using the Finite Element Method (FEM) was performed to the links and shafts assembled as in Figure 14 to verify stress state and resistance for different load conditions, then new dimensions were defined for the mechanism to comply with admissible stresses on the different materials. The analysis was achieved using SolidWorks® 2012. For the assembly contact without penetration was considered between surfaces, this type of connection prevents interference between the components in contact, allowing the formation of gaps, i.e., permits relative movement between the components. All simulations were static, with linear and isotropic materials as shown in Table 2.

Table 2. Material properties for different components. Taken from [23,27]

Components	Links	Axes
Material	Aluminum 7075 T6	Stainless steel 304
Young modulus (GPa)	72	200
Poisson modulus	0.33	0.3
Yield strength (MPa)	503	241
Ultimate strength (MPa)	572	586

All components were meshed using a 10 nodes parabolic tetrahedral solid element. Convergence analysis was done considering maximum von Mises stress, strain and equivalent strain energy. Three different load conditions were studied as follows:

- Load condition 1: specifications established by the standard ISO 10328 [4] were used for the main structural test, specifically the maximum load condition I, corresponding to the initial stage of the stance phase of the gait cycle, near the instant where the heel contact occurs.
- Load condition 2: also with the specifications of the standard ISO 10328 [4], but for maximum load condition II, associated with the final stage of the support phase of gait cycle, close to the toe take off towards the swing phase.
- Load condition 3: the prosthesis is subjected to a compression force of 1,000 N (equal to the weight of a one leg standing person 100 kg), load was located as a pressure on the top link of the device.

Figure 16 shows the specifications for the ISO 10328 detailing the location of the loads and Table 3 shows the magnitude and geometric distances corresponding to each load condition.

Figure 17 shows the configuration of load I (F=2,240 N), which is remote in relation to the prosthetic knee. The coronal plane is observed in Figure 17a, marked distances refer to 'O_K=50mm' and 'O_B=45mm' for loading condition I, as indicated in Table 3; Figure 17b shows the sagittal plane with distances 'f_K=52mm' and 'f_B=48mm'. Figure 17c presents the boundary conditions where the movement of the top surface of upper link was restricted to zero while a compression load was applied on the bottom surface of lower link.

Table 3. ISO 10328: magnitude and geometric distances for each load condition. Taken from [4]

	Load Condition I	Load Condition II
Load Mag. (N)	2,240	2,013
f_K (mm)	52	72
o_K (mm)	-50	-35
f_B (mm)	-48	129
o_B (mm)	45	-19
u_K - u_B (mm)	500	500

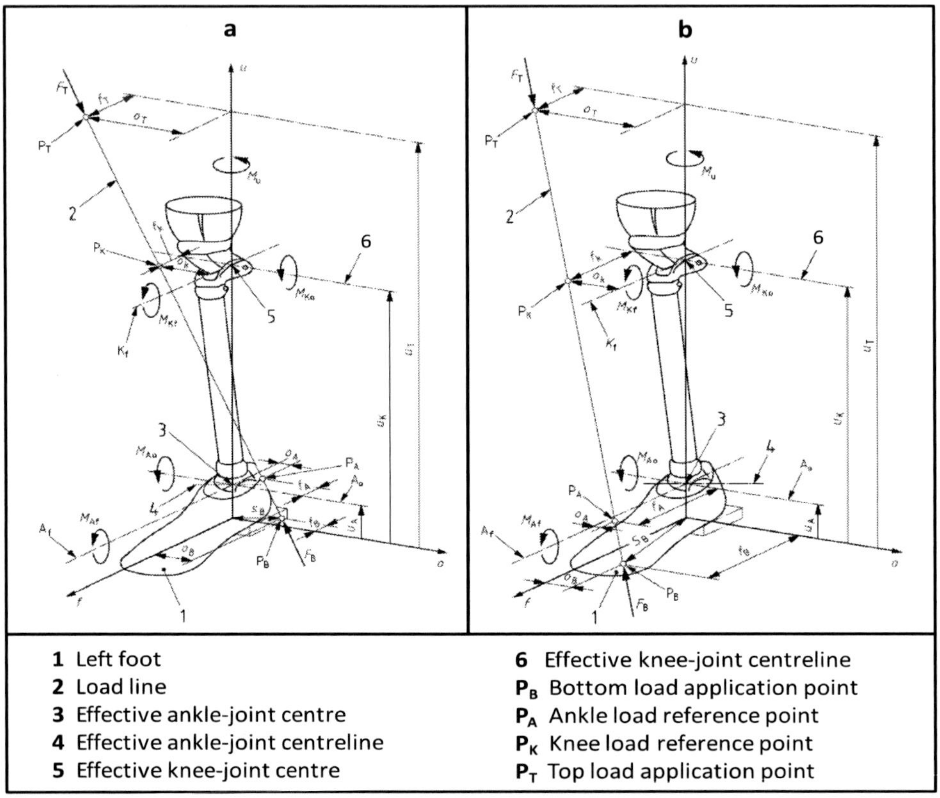

Figure 16. ISO 10328, static resistance test: (a) Maximum load condition I, (b) Maximum load condition II (taken and adapted from [4]).

Figure 18 shows the meshed model for the loading conditions tested; for the load case 1, most critical loading condition, the model converged for 90,091 elements.

The analyses results show a 647.41 MPa maximum von Mises stress that occurs in the lower part of link ‘a’ observable in Figure 19, close to the contact zone of the link ‘a’ with the link ‘d’. Detailing the maximum stress value on each component (see Table 4) is to be noticed that link ‘d’ is also subjected to high stresses, with a maximum value of 622.83 MPa. With respect to the axes, the upper rear axis is the most demanded one, with a maximum stress of 455.07 MPa, followed by the upper front axis with 327.72 MPa. Figure 20 shows the results obtained for the load case 2, the maximum von Mises stress is 475.98 MPa and occurs in the link 'd' at one end of the extension stop surface. Table 4 shows the maximum von Mises stress for each component for all three load cases.

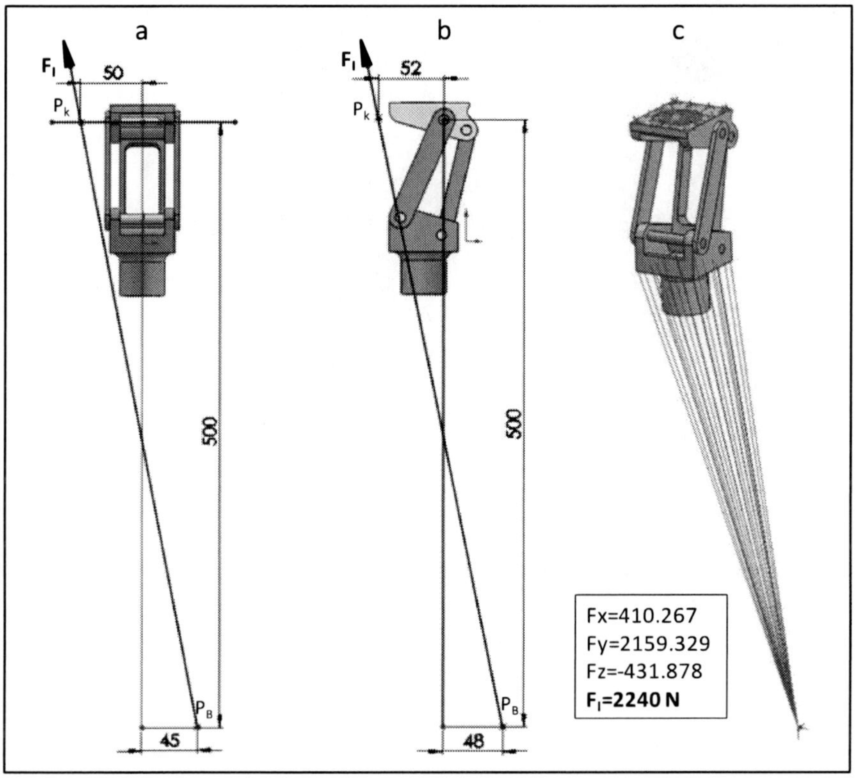

Figure 17. Configuration of the load condition I according to the ISO 10238.

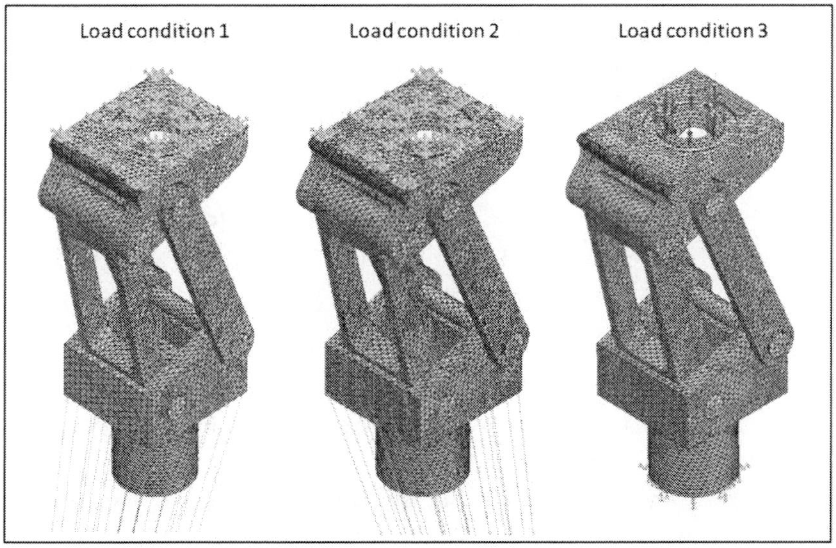

Figure 18. Meshed model for loading conditions studied.

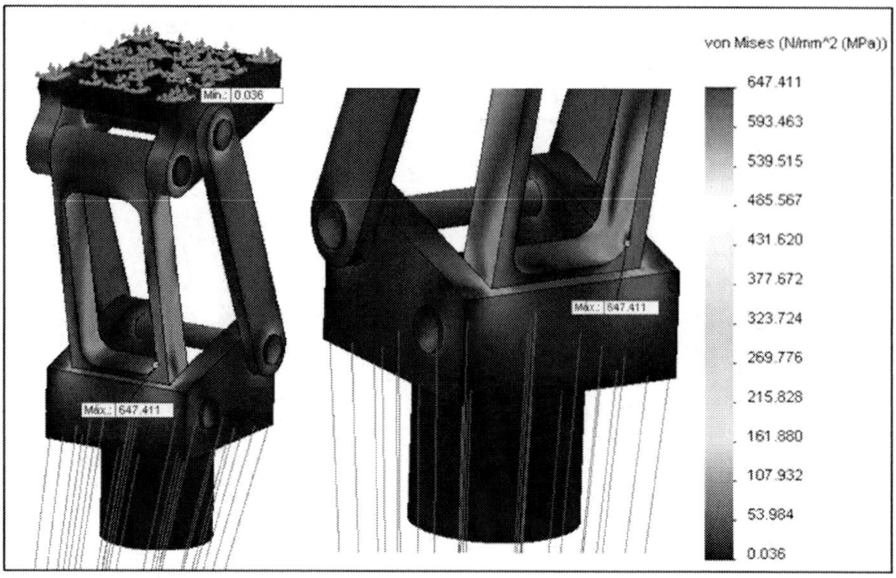

Figure 19. von Mises stress distribution of the mechanism for load condition 1.

Considering that the structural design requires that all safety factors must be above 1, and the results shown in Table 4 indicate that safety factors of links 'a' and 'd' and upper front and rear axes are below 1, redesigning these components was mandatory. At the same time, an optimal design was also pursued for reducing the weight as much as possible.

Table 4. Maximum von Mises stress and safety factor for each component of the prosthesis for the three load cases

	Condition 1		Condition 2		Condition 3	
Component	Max. Stress (MPa)	Safety factor	Max. Stress (MPa)	Safety factor	Max. Stress (MPa)	Safety factor
Link a	647.41	0.78	417.15	1.21	119.78	4.20
Link b	458.77	1.10	432.28	1.16	104.64	4.81
Link c1	330.08	1.52	420.19	1.20	96.68	5.20
Link c2	486.25	1.03	423.07	1.19	91.85	5.48
Link d	622.83	0.81	475.98	1.06	133.11	3.78
Upper front axis	327.72	0.74	314.84	0.77	77.91	3.09
Upper rear axis	455.07	0.53	411.49	0.59	109.20	2.21
Lower front axis	240.92	1.00	309.33	0.78	46.06	5.23
Lower rear axis	192.43	1.25	185.38	1.30	39.94	6.03

To raise the safety factor at the mentioned critical components the following changes were introduced: increase of the diameters of the upper and lower front axes from 8 mm to 10 mm, increase of the rear upper arms width from 8 mm to 11 mm, increase of the extension stop thickness of link 'd', increase of dimensions of the link 'a', reinforcement of the areas close to the axes holes of links 'c1' and 'c2'. Once such changes were applied, new stress analyses showed that all components of the prosthesis reached a safety factor greater than 1 for all load cases. Figure 21b shows the redesigned prosthesis.

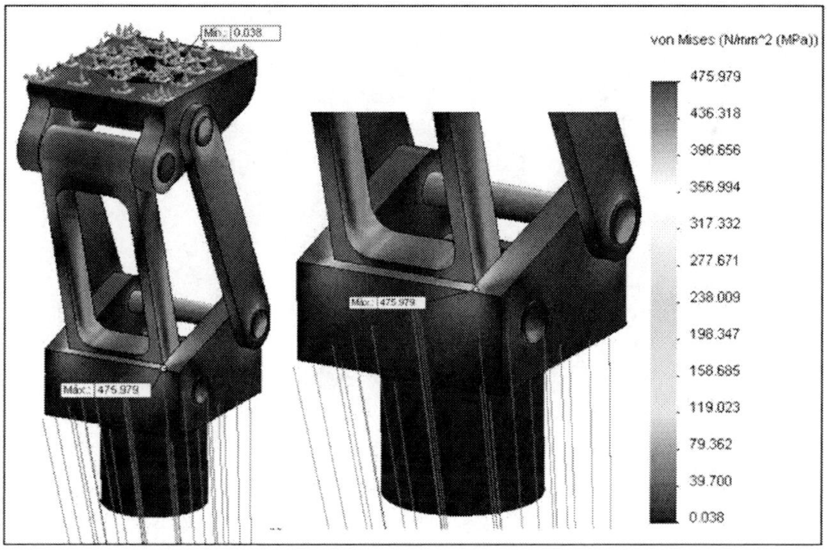

Figure 20. von Mises stress distribution of the mechanism for load condition 2.

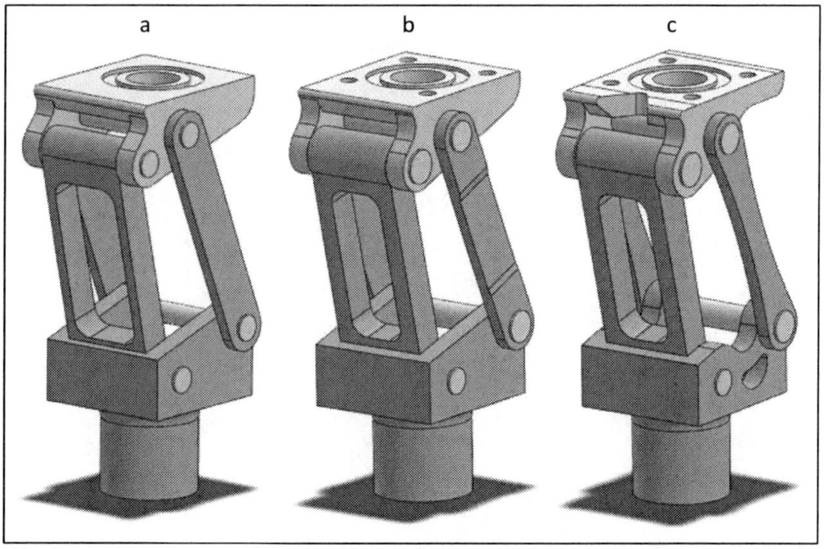

Figure 21. Polycentric knee prosthesis: (a) Initial model, (b) Redesigned model, (c) Rectified model.

Subsequently, taking into account the results of stress analyses of the redesigned prosthesis and with the aim of decreasing mass, further modifications on some parts of the prosthesis were done intervening areas of low stresses; specifically, changes in the links ‘b’, ‘c1’, ‘c2’ and ‘d’ were performed as detailed in Figure 21c. Finally, a last stress analysis (including convergence analysis) was carried out and results yielded a safety factor above 1 for all components and all load cases (see Table 5). Figure 22 shows the results for the load case 1.

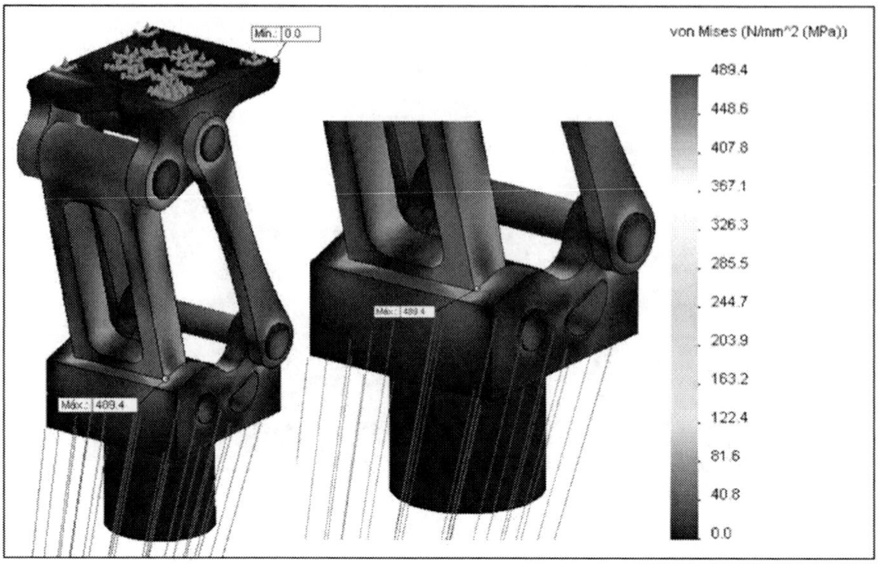

Figure 22. von Mises stress distribution of the rectified mechanism for load condition 1.

Table 5. Maximum von Mises stress and safety factor for each component of the rectified prosthesis for the three load cases

Component	Condition 1 Max. Stress (MPa)	Condition 1 Safety factor	Condition 2 Max. Stress (MPa)	Condition 2 Safety factor	Condition 3 Max. Stress (MPa)	Condition 3 Safety factor
Link a	413.92	1.22	223.01	2.26	82.24	6.12
Link b	365.09	1.38	276.34	1.82	69.64	7.22
Link c1	250.96	2.00	381.58	1.32	63.93	7.87
Link c2	395.58	1.27	365.52	1.38	65.00	7.74
Link d	489.4	1.03	363.57	1.38	106.81	4.71
Upper front axis	220.91	1.09	220.72	1.09	41.63	5.79
Upper rear axis	222.31	1.08	200.83	1.20	40.67	5.93
Lower front axis	142.01	1.70	230.01	1.05	31.15	7.74
Lower rear axis	174.92	1.38	167.1	1.44	36.29	6.64

2.2.3. Design of Assistant Extension Mechanism

A mechanism for assisting extension was also included in the prosthesis design, among its functions there are limiting the flexion angle of the knee, providing smooth forward swinging of the distal portion of the prosthesis during the swing phase and forcing the prosthetic knee to reach full extension easily and without producing a final impact. As aforementioned, in polycentric mechanisms the center of rotation of the knee is not fixed and therefore, the lever arm for extension has a significant variation with knee flexion angle. A schematic draw (see Figure 23) shows the force line of the AEM with respect to the ICR and moment arm R_c.

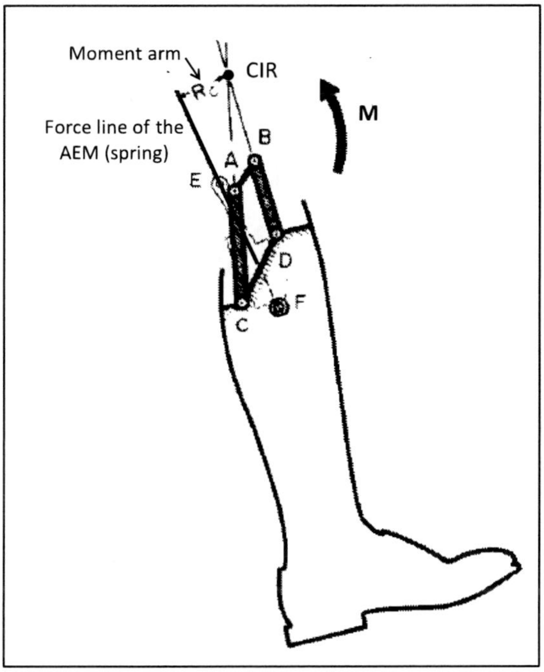

Figure 23. Extension moment of a polycentric knee prosthesis (adapted from [28]).

A spring with fixed stiffness constant was selected as the basis for the extension mechanism. This is a low cost and easy to assemble system that meets the requirements of mobility meant in the conceptual design. For the design was necessary:

- Brain storming and evaluation of different proposals over the AEM configuration and location.
- Selection of spring characteristics and properties.
- Calculation of moment arm of spring action line respect to ICR for each knee flexion angle.
- Estimation of knee extension moment required, considering full range of prosthesis flexion.
- Design of parts for installation of spring in the prosthesis.

After evaluating several proposals for developing the AEM, the one shown in Figure 24a was selected. The compression spring was located internally in the structure of the prosthesis, specifically between bottom link 'd' and rear link 'a'. This configuration ensures effective and linear compression of the spring with knee flexion and eases installation.

Regarding the compression spring, it was decided to evaluate multiple compression springs available commercially. The following springs characteristics were measured: free length, total number of active coils, outer and inner diameters of the spring and wire diameter. The springs constants were obtained experimentally with an universal testing machine and the shear modulus of the material of the spring was calculated. The physical dimensions of the final spring and its parameters are presented in Table 6.

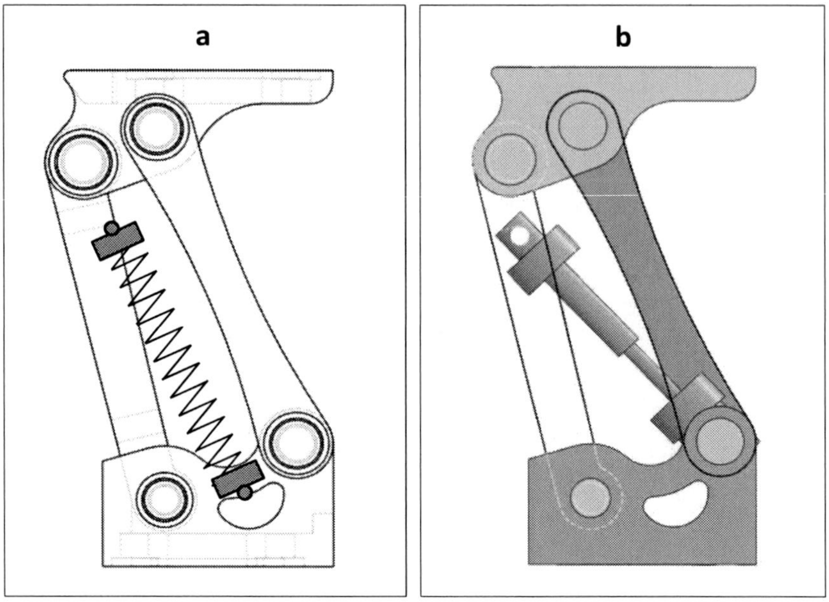

Figure 24. Proposal selected for: (a) Compression spring to assist extension, (b) Installation of the resulting AEM.

To define location of the AEM within the prosthesis, the moment of extension produced for each knee flexion angle was primarily valued, considering the moment arm of the spring force line in relation to the ICR of the mechanism. To avoid resistance during the first 15° of knee flexion during the gait cycle, the extension moment should be small, and then from 20 to 65°, during swing phase, it should increase to ensure full extension before heel strike. It is also necessary to guarantee very small extension moment, close to zero (0), for flexion angles greater than 80°, in order that during sitting (flexion to 90°) or maximum flexion (131.5°) knee does not extend involuntarily.

Table 6. Physical dimensions of the final spring and calculated parameters

Parameter	Spring 1	Spring 2
Outer diameter (Do) [mm]	14.5	10
Inner diameter (Di) [mm]	10.5	7
Wire diameter (dw) [mm]	2.0	1.5
Free lenght (Lf) [mm]	76	87
Total number of coils (Nt)	18	28
End types	Closed, squared and ground	Closed, squared and ground
Number of active coils (Na)	16	26
Elastic constant (K) [N/mm]	4.51	1.61
Average diameter (Dm) [mm]	12.5	8.5
Turn length [mm]	4.50	3.23
Shear modulus of the material (G) [GPa]	70.59	40.68

The selected proposal for installation (Figure 24b) required minimal changes in the structure of the prosthesis; the upper spring support is fitted on a pin located on the rear link ‘a’ of the prosthesis while the lower spring support is directly on the lower front axis. In

Figure 25, it is observed location of the spring load arm for flexion angles of 0, 20, 40 and 90°.

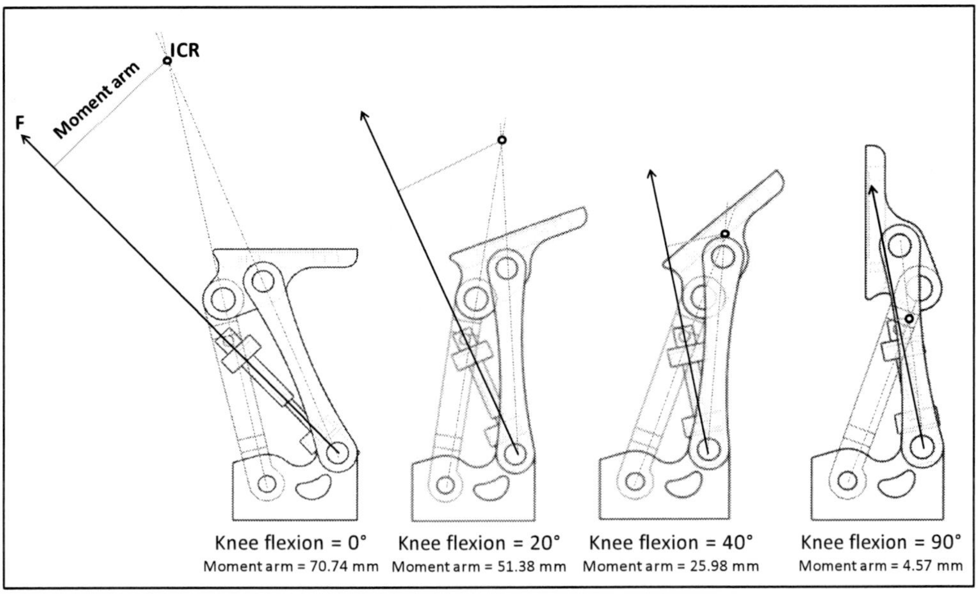

Figure 25. Moment arm for flexion angles of 0, 20, 40 and 90°.

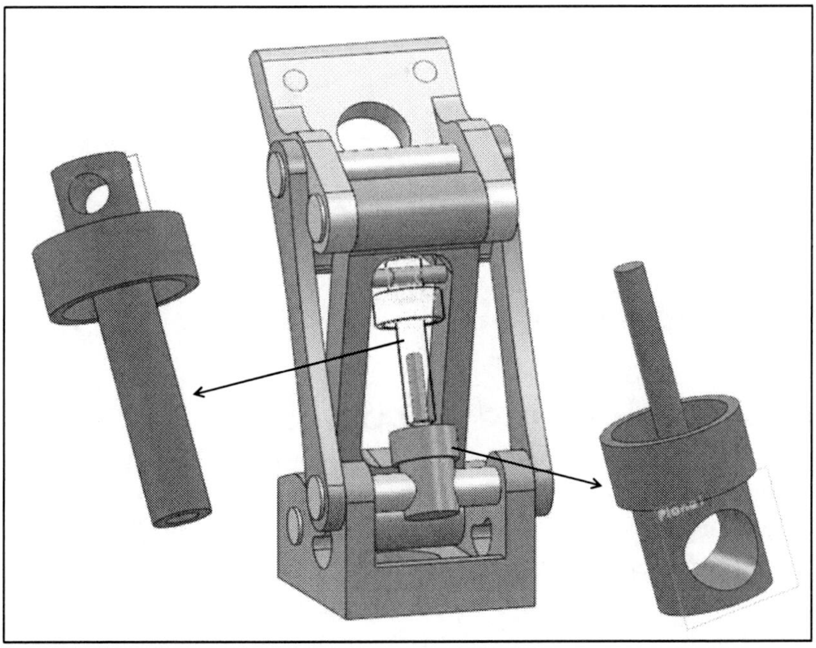

Figure 26. Brackets designed for placement of the AEM on the prosthesis.

To design the parts for installation of spring in the prosthesis, Mott [27] considerations were taken into account; he notes that to install a spring in a cylindrical hole, or around a rod, adequate clearances should be provided as diameter increases while compressing the spring.

To prevent rubbing, for diameters of 12 mm or greater, the hole diametrical clearance must be one tenth of spring wire diameter. In this regard, two configurations for assisting extension were considered, first, installation of only one spring, and second, use of two springs in parallel where one is located inside the other (see Figure 26).

To install the spring in the first configuration it was necessary to modify its free length, the final spring length was 61 mm and its new spring constant was 5.56 N/mm. Figure 27 shows extension moment versus knee flexion angle for this configuration. For this setting at 0° flexion, moment is 1.57 N.m and maximum (5.02 N.m) occurs at 20° of flexion; at 60° moment is 1.91 N.m and at 90° it is very small, 0.62 N.m, until reaching 0 N.m at 120°. For the second configuration, two springs were used with length 61 mm, whereby the spring constant were 5.56 N/mm for spring 1 and 2.32 N/mm for spring 2. Figure 27 also shows the extension moment curves versus knee flexion angle for this second configuration. Both graphs are similar, but with different magnitudes; the idea is to use the more convenient arrangement (one or two springs) depending on the patient's requirements.

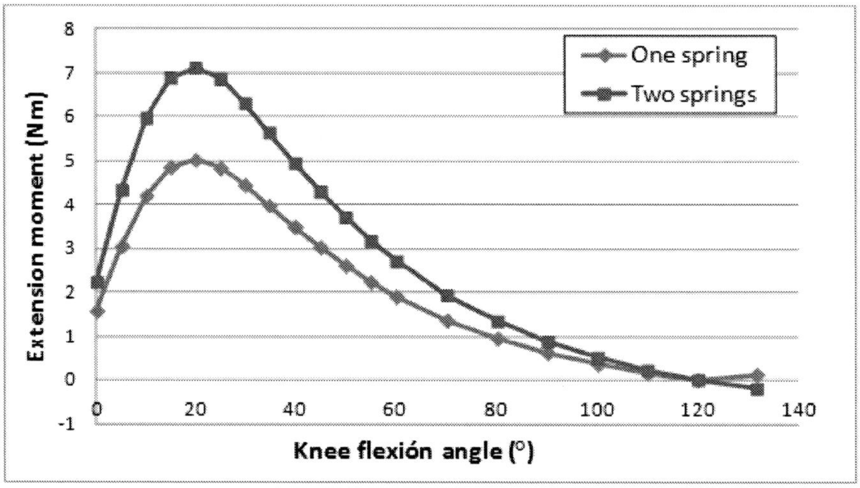

Figure 27. Extension moment versus knee flexion angle for: (a) configuration using one spring, (b) configuration using two springs in parallel.

3. Manufacturing and Assembly of the Prosthesis

In total 5 links, 4 axes, 14 bushings and 4 springs supports were manufactured. The links were manufactured on a Computer Numerical Control (CNC) milling machine, starting from the STL CAD files models of each piece, obtained from SolidWorks®; the geometry of the parts and the required precision were decisive criteria for using the CNC. The other components were manufactured combining conventional lathe and milling machine; Figure 28 shows the assembled prosthesis.

For testing the PKM manufactured, as part of an entire assembly of a lower limb prosthesis for transfemoral amputees (see Figure 29), the assistance of a qualified prosthetist was required. He performed both static and dynamic alignments on volunteer patients to test the prosthesis.

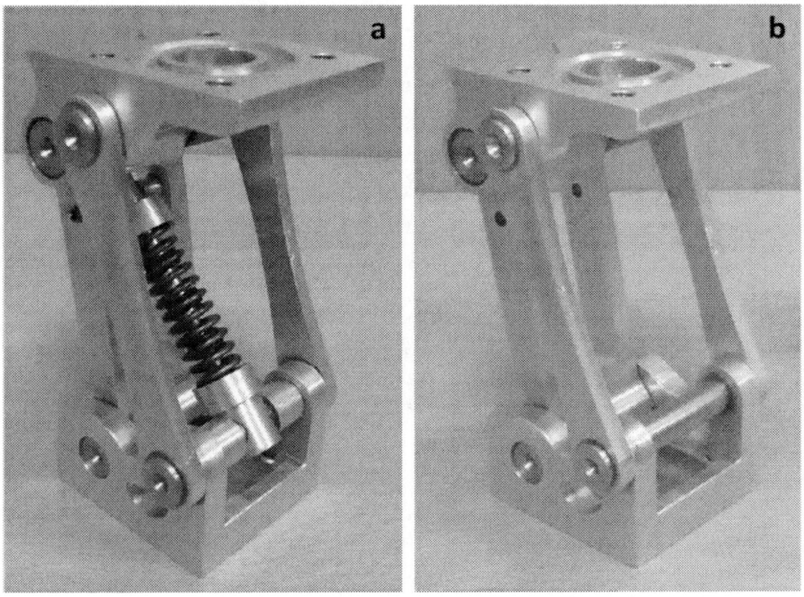

Figura 28. (a) Manufactured and assembled prosthesis, (b) Assembled prosthesis with AEM.

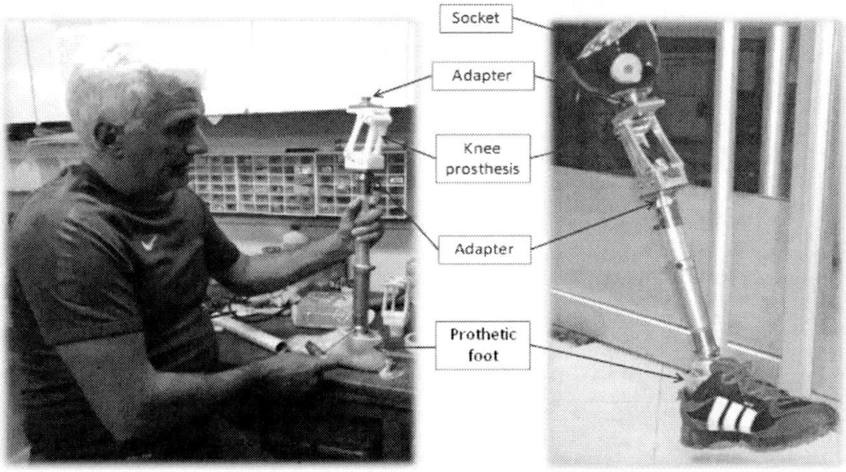

Figure 29. Entire assembly of a lower limb prosthesis for transfemoral amputees.

4. Prosthesis Testing

In order to verify the adjustments and analyze preliminary performance of the developed prosthesis (from now on USB prosthesis), four different test were performed: 1) prosthesis worn by a normal individual without amputation by means of a custom-made simulator on a treadmill, 2) preliminary test with a transfemoral amputee patient wearing the prosthesis, 3) clinical gait analysis on two patients with transfemoral amputation, and 4) comparative analysis regarding the prosthesis Otto Bock 3R20.

4.1. Test with Prosthesis Simulator

The objective of this test was to verify structural stability of the prosthesis under walking loads, as well as functioning of the PKM before placing the AEM; particularly to evaluate the behavior of the former during balance towards full extension before starting the next stride. The test was performed using a simulator socket for a normal leg in 90° of flexion, available by one of the co-authors, as shown in Figure 30. The test was carried out walking on a treadmill at different speeds.

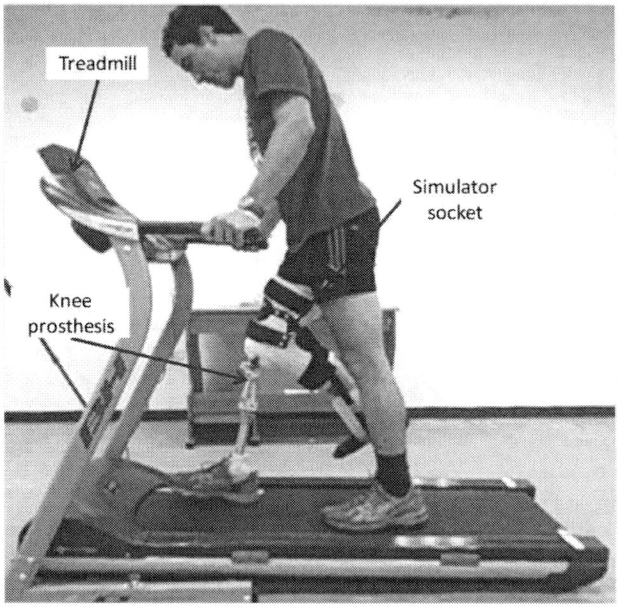

Figure 30. Co-author testing the prosthesis using a simulator on a treadmill at different speeds.

The results showed structural stability of the prosthesis, however, during low speed tests the prosthesis did not extend completely at the end of the swing phase, making difficult the proper heel contact to initiate the next stride; Figure 30 shows the flexion of the prosthetic knee during initial contact. This behavior confirmed the need to install the AEM previously described, which was installed for the next testing, at the same time detected friction between some links was also corrected.

4.2. Test with Transfemoral Amputee

The prosthesis was tested by patient 1 of Table 7 after signed informed consent. The tests were conducted under the supervision of a qualified prosthetist on the premises of an orthopaedics facility. The prosthetist performed the installation of the device on the patient and carried out static and dynamic alignments (see Figure 31). The objective of this test was to verify the overall functioning of the prosthesis and get the feedback of both patient and prosthetist.

Table 7. Patients with transfemoral amputation

Description	Patients	
	Patient 1	Patient 2
Amputation	Left (unilateral)	Right (unilateral)
Sex	Masculine	Masculine
Age	23 years	21 years
Weight	85 kg	79 kg
Height	173.5 cm	171 cm
Prosthesis use experience	6 year	18 month

The patient began the gait on the parallel bars and after several excursions, he considered safe to undertake corridors of the premises, driving the prosthesis under different trials in forward motion, with all body weight support, lateral flexion displacement, lateral displacement in full extension, rearward displacement, and maximum flexion during the pendulum movement (see Figure 32). The outcomes obtained from the patient's opinion and observational analysis of prosthetist and authors included: structural stability of the prosthesis during normal walking, walking backwards and sideways movements; correct flexion during walking or sitting position; and correct extension after rolling.

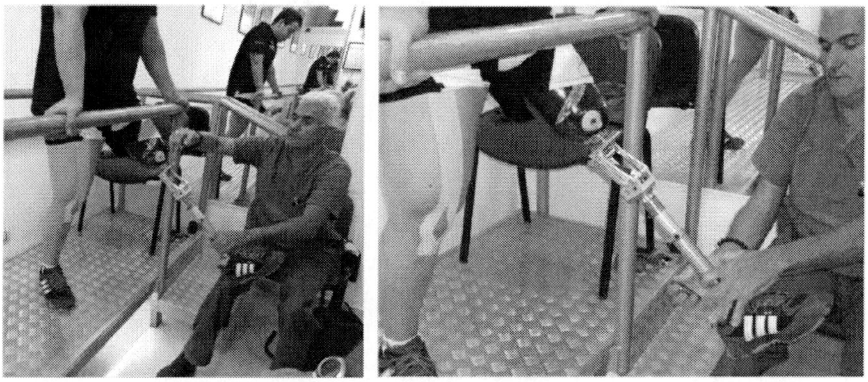

Figure 31. Positioning and alignment of the prosthesis to patient 1.

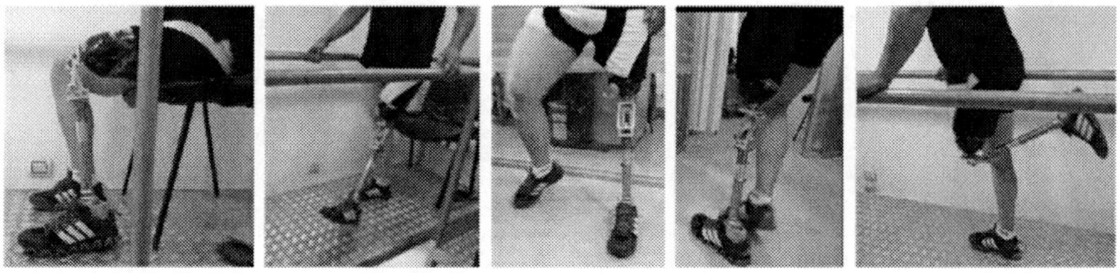

Figure 32. Preliminary test of the prosthesis on patient 1.

4.3. Gait Analysis of Transfemoral Amputees Wearing the USB Prosthesis

Two patients with unilateral transfemoral amputation (described in Table 7) tested the USB prosthesis at the Center for Motion Analysis of the Simón Bolívar University (CAM-

USB). Measurements for kinematics (flexion/extension of the hip, knee and ankle) and kinetics (moment and power of hip, knee and ankle) in the sagittal plane for lower body were taken. Reflective markers were placed in patients using the Helen Hayes protocol [20], data was acquired at a sampling frequency of 100 fps and was processed using the Cortex® software from MotionAnalysis Corp. The tests included multiple trails at self-selected speed; adaptation time of patients with prosthesis was an hour prior to testing. Figure 33 show patients using the USB prosthesis with reflective markers placed on lower limbs landmarks.

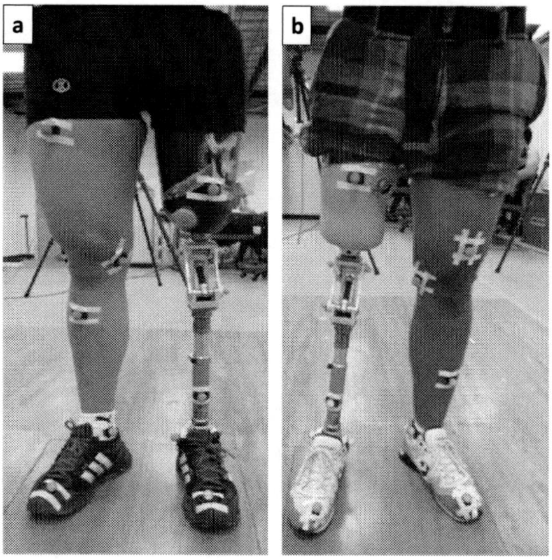

Figure 33. (a) Patient 1 with USB prosthesis, (b) Patient 2 with USB prosthesis.

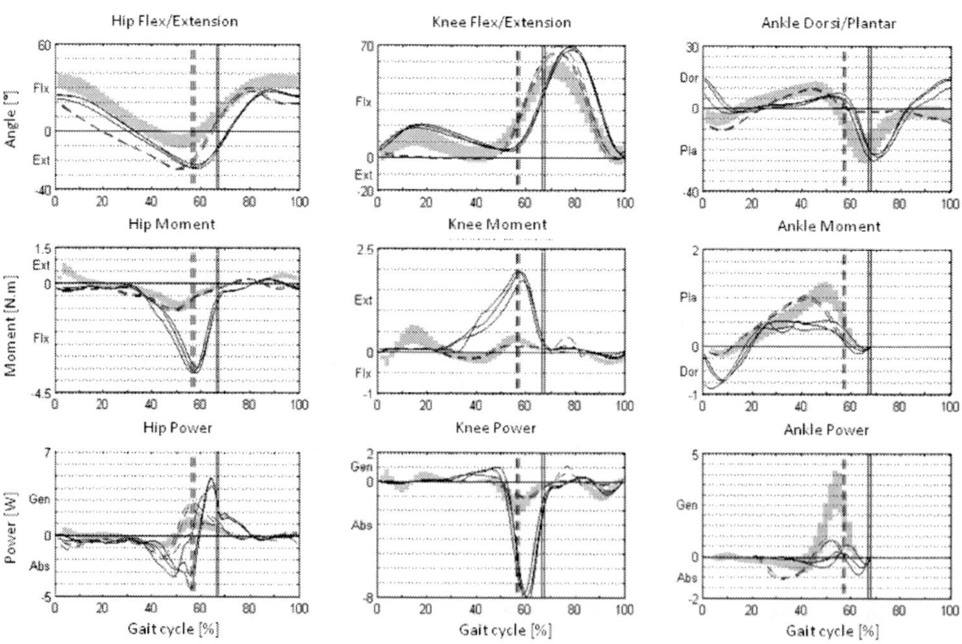

Figure 34. Kinematics and kinetics of hip, knee and ankle for healthy leg (continuous line) and prosthetic leg (dashed line) of patient 1 wearing the USB knee prosthesis.

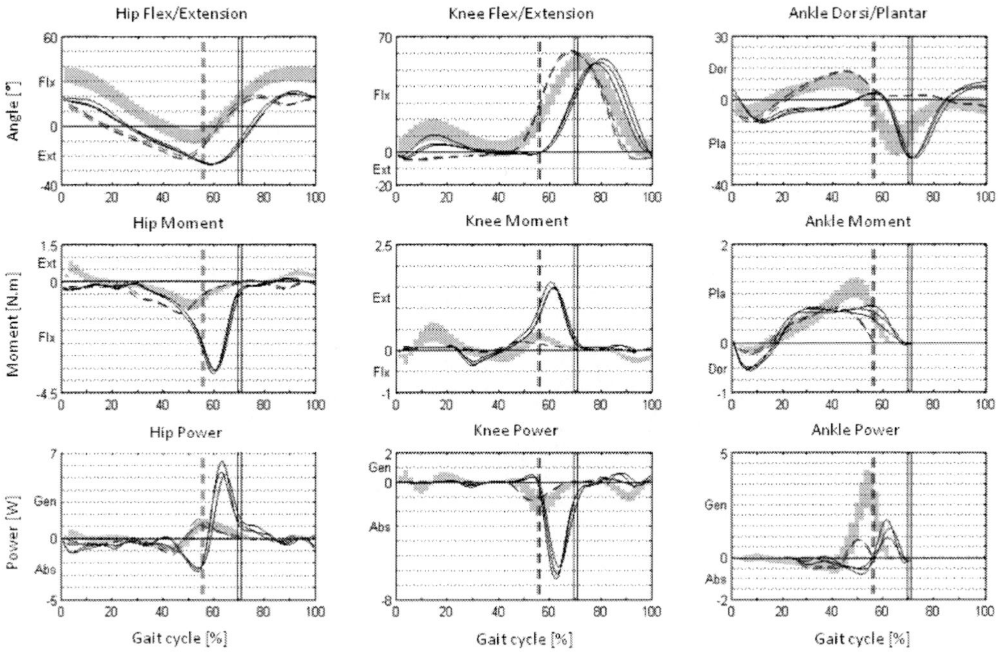

Figure 35. Kinematics and kinetics of hip, knee and ankle for healthy leg (continuous line) and prosthetic leg (dashed line) of patient 2 wearing the USB knee prosthesis.

Table 8. Spatio-temporal variables from patients 1 and 2 using the USB prosthesis

	USB prosthesis	Speed (m/s)	Stride length (m)	Cadence (stride/min)	% stance
Patient 1	Sound limb	1.24	1.38	110.8	67.3
	Prosthetic limb	1.24	1.37	110.8	56.1
Patient 2	Sound limb	1.09	1.30	104.2	69.9
	Prosthetic limb	1.09	1.31	104.2	54.7

Kinematics and kinetics of hip, knee and ankle (Figure 34) and spatio-temporal variables (Table 8) of patient 1 using the USB prosthesis follow the typical behavior of transfemoral amputees gait with respect to a normal pattern (gray stripe).

More in detail, knee flexion achieved by the prosthetic leg in the swing phase is close to normal, however flexion during the support phase (0 to 50% of the gait cycle) is approximately 0°, which agrees with what has been reported by other authors on gait of transfemoral amputees [21]. For the prosthetic leg after the stance phase (60% of the gait cycle) no plantar flexion occurs, the ankle flexion angle becomes practically 0° and constant throughout the balance, this result coincides with that obtained by [29]. The kinematics of the healthy leg has a similar behavior to the reference curves of people without pathologies in their lower limbs, though an important compensatory activity is observed regarding the kinetics of knee and hip; this coincides with that reported by [30] and [31]. The duration of stance phase of gait cycle of the healthy leg was greater than the prosthetic one, which comes from the natural confidence felt by the patient in his healthy leg, therefore keeping it longer in contact with the floor. Similar results were obtained on patient 2 (Figure 35 and Table 8).

4.3.1. Comparative Analysis of Performance of the USB Prosthesis Relative to the Otto Bock 3R20 Prosthesis

In order to compare the USB prosthesis performance in relation to other commercial prostheses, we performed a comparative gait analysis study. Everyday knee prosthesis of patient 1 was the Otto Bock 3R80 (monocentric prosthesis with rotational hydraulic system), though he also used the Otto Bock 3R78 (4-bar polycentric pneumatic control mechanism for swing phase).

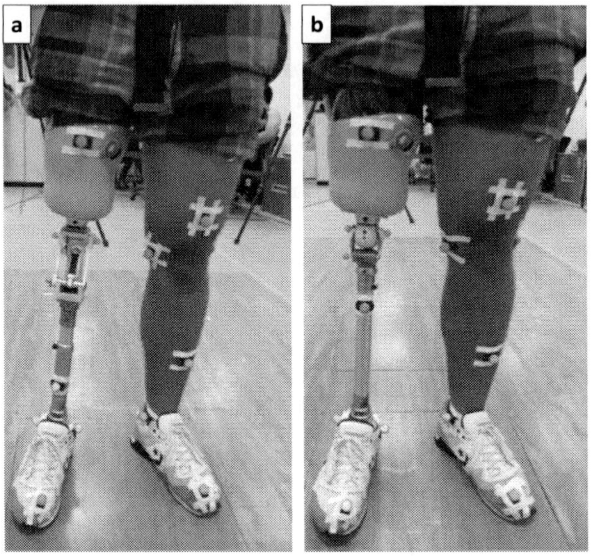

Figure 36. Patient 2 using: (a) USB prosthesis, (b) Otto Bock 3R20 prosthesis.

Everyday prosthesis of patient 2 was the Otto Bock 3R20 (4-bar polycentric mechanical knee with a compression spring to assist the extension).

The characteristics of the Otto Bock 3R20 prosthesis makes it directly comparable with the USB prosthesis, therefore a comparative performance biomechanical study with patient 2 using the Otto Bock 3R20 and the USB prosthesis was conducted. Kinematics in the sagittal plane, as well as kinetics of hip, knee and ankle, and the space-time variables for both legs were measured and compared. Figure 36 shows patient 2 using both devices.

Results shown in Figure 37 and Figure 38 indicate that kinematics and kinetics of hip, knee and ankle, from both prostheses are very similar, existing overlap in most curves, including kinetic knee and hip compensatory activity of the sound leg (relative to the reference). Patient spatio-temporal variables (Table 9) show some differences however: stride length and cadence (of the sound and prosthetic leg) are 4.8% and 13.3% higher for the USB prosthesis compared to the 3R20 respectively.

The prosthetic leg support percentage when using the USB prosthesis is slightly larger than when using the 3R20, while the percentage support of the sound leg is slightly smaller; this indicates a favorable performance of the USB prosthesis, which is reflected in a decrement of the asymmetry between sound and prosthetic limbs.

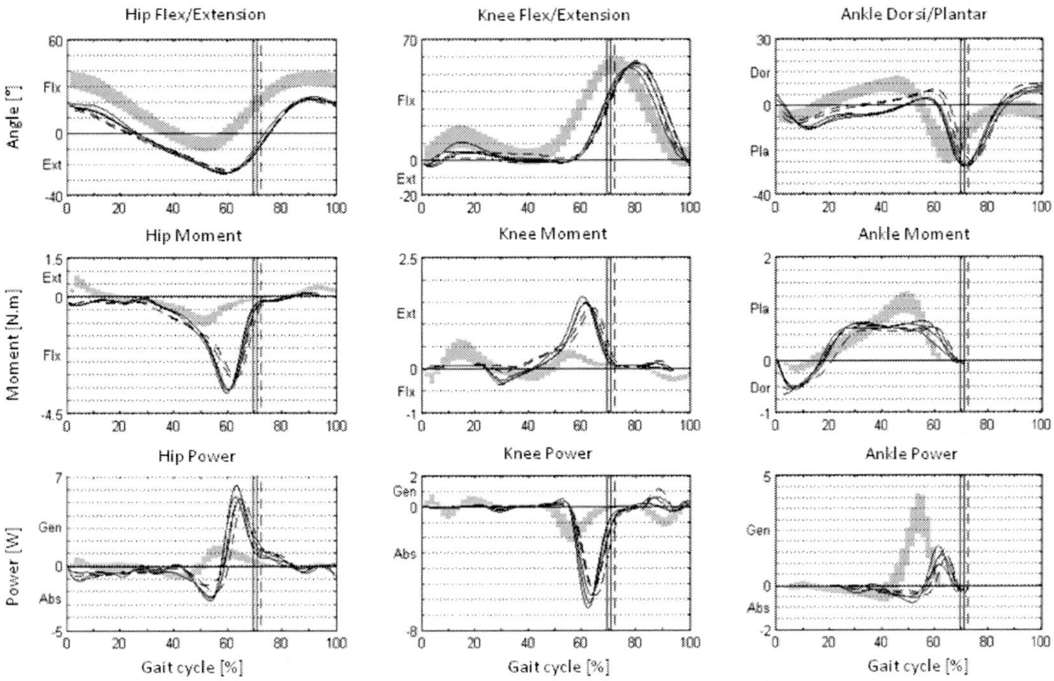

Figure 37. Kinematics and kinetics of hip, knee and ankle of patient 2 for sound limb using USB prostheses (continuous line) and Otto Bock 3R20 (dashed line).

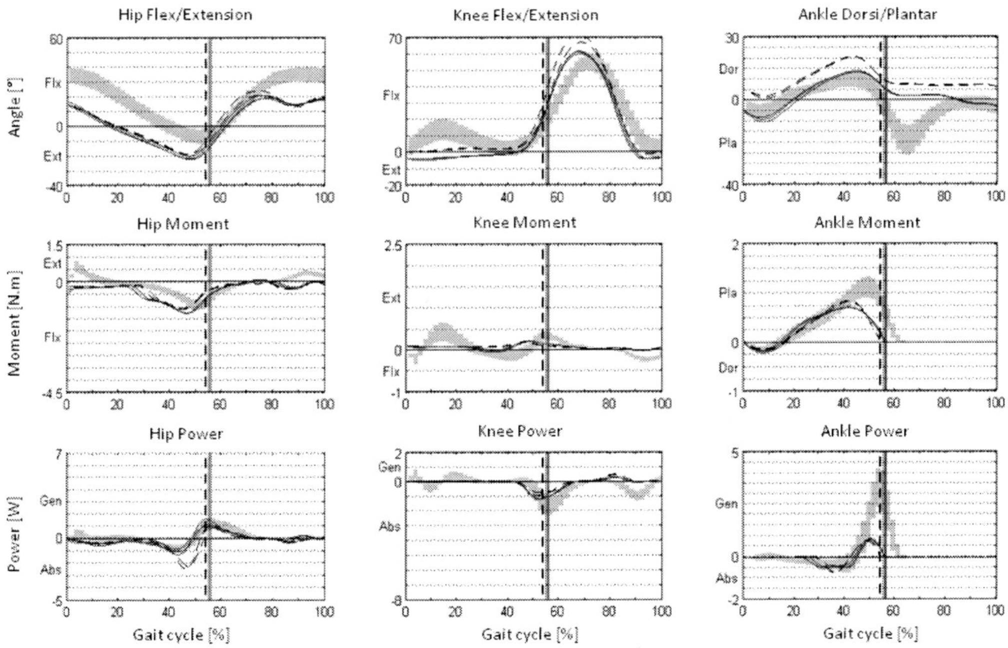

Figure 38. Kinematics and kinetics of hip, knee and ankle of patient 2 for prosthetic limb using prostheses USB (continuous line) and Otto Bock 3R20 (dashed line).

Table 9. Patient 2: Spatio-temporal variables using prostheses USB and Otto Bock 3R20

	Patient 2	Speed (m/s)	Stride length (m)	Cadence (stride/min)	% stance
USB prosthesis	Sound limb	1.09	1.30	104.2	69.9
	Prosthetic limb	1.09	1.31	104.2	54.7
Otto Bock 3R20	Sound limb	0.97	1.24	92.0	71.2
	Prosthetic limb	0.97	1.25	92.0	53.3

Conclusion

A mechanical knee prosthesis was developed considering safety, functionality and cost as the most important variables for conceptual design, responding the needs of transfemoral amputees in Venezuela. Particularly, a 4-bar polycentric mechanism was the device selected for carry out the design of details. The methodology used in this research decanted into an original proposal for a knee prosthesis, which involved dimensioning of the mechanism considering the optimal kinematic behavior, structural analysis and ease to assist extension. The definition of the 6 parameters that configure the mechanism was solved using a genetic algorithm within an iterative process, which additionally involved a tailor-developed computing platform that integrated data obtained from gait analysis and equations governing kinematic of the mechanism.

The structural design yielded a device capable to support severe loading conditions. Stress analysis, using the Finite Element Method, was performed following the specification of the ISO 10328. During the design of the mechanism to assist extension, the location of ICR for each flexion angle was crucial; particularly to determine the variable moment of extension and the necessary spring force. The compression spring was located internally in the structure of the prosthesis, guaranteeing effective linear spring deformation with knee flexion, straightforward installation and minor modifications in the structure of the prosthesis. The mechanism designed effectively limits the sudden knee flexion and forces full extension right before next heel strike.

The manufacture of the prosthesis was done using conventional lathe, which ensures low cost of production to the benefit of future users. Through observational analysis was possible to verify the structural stability of the device during free test, as well as the correct flexion and extension during walking or sitting position. Clinical gait analyses done to two patients showed that both kinematics and kinetics of prosthetic and sound legs are similar to those referenced in the literature for amputee patients. Moreover the kinematic and kinetic results were comparable with the behavior of the commercial prosthesis Otto Bock 3R20; indeed, gait speed using the USB prosthesis was slightly higher than with the latter, presenting even a decrease in the asymmetric characteristic of gait between both sides in patients with unilateral amputation.

Finally, we can say that the prosthesis guarantees desired performance during gait, including knee stability after heel strike and during loading response, and voluntary flexion during terminal stance and before pre-swing.

Acknowledgments

The authors gratefully acknowledge the contribution of C. P. O. Fernando Carvalho, for his assistance in the fitting and alignment of the prosthesis, as well to all the personnel of his workshop BIOTECPRO, C. A. Also, we are deeply grateful to Mr. Frank Ávila and Mr. Edgar Burgos, for offering themselves as volunteers to test the prosthesis during the development of this project.

This project is currently being funded by the Project No. PEI-2147 of the National Fund for Science, Innovation and Technology of Venezuela.

References

[1] Radcliffe, C. W. (1994). Four-bar linkage prosthetic knee mechanisms: kinematics, alignment and prescription criteria. *Prosthetics and Orthotics, Vol. 18*, pp. 159-173.

[2] Amador, B. T., Müller-Karger, C. M., Casanova, E. & Torrealba, R. R. (2013). Structural analysis during the design of polycentric prosthetic knee. Proceedings of the 14th Congress of the International Society of Biomechanics ISB'2013, Natal-Brazil, pp. 42.

[3] Amador, B. T., Müller-Karger, C. M., Torrealba, R. R. & Vidal, A. (2013). Comparación de las condiciones de contacto en el análisis estructural de una prótesis policéntrica de rodilla. Proceedings of the Panamerican Health Care Exchanges Conference PAHCE'2013, Medellin-Colombia, pp. 60-65.

[4] ISO 10328. Prosthetics – Structural testing of lower-limb prostheses – Requirements and test methods. 1st Edition. ISO; 2006.

[5] Carvalho, J. Amputacões de membros inferiores. Em busca da plena reabilitacaõ. 2nd Edition. Brasil: Manole; 2003.

[6] Alós Villacrosa, J. Amputaciones del miembro inferior en cirugía vascular. 1st Edition. Barcelona: Editorial Glosa; 2008.

[7] Gard, S., Childress, D. & Uellendahi, J. (1996). The influence of four-bar linkage knees on prosthetic swing-phase floor clearance. *Journal of Prosthetics and Orthotics, Vol. 8, No. 2*, pp. 34-40.

[8] Michael, J. W. (1999). Modern prosthetic knee mechanisms. *Clinical Orthopaedics and Related Research, No. 361*, pp. 39-47.

[9] DAW Industries. Technical Report on the TGK-5PS0SLK, TGK-5PS0 and TGK-50S0 PC Knee Units. San Diego-USA: Department of Research and Development; 1997.

[10] González Rico, M. Pediatric knee project CIREC. Masters thesis (not published). Bogotá-Colombia: Universidad de Los Andes; 2005.

[11] Correal, S., Palacio, L. & Salázar, I. (2006). Análisis FEA de prótesis de rodilla policéntrica (FEA analysis of polycentric knee prosthesis). *Avances en Sistemas e Informática, Vol. 3, No. 1*, pp. 35-38.

[12] Enríquez, J., Alonso, E., Méndez, A. & Pérez, L. (2007). Diseño y construcción de una prótesis de rodilla con pistón magnetoreológico. Proceedings of the 8th Congreso Iberoamericano de Ingeniería Mecánica, Cusco-Perú.

[13] Valentino, G., Guerrero, L., Obregón, D. & Avalos, O. (2008). Desarrollo de prótesis externa de rodilla con mecanismo policéntrico (Development of external knee prosthesis with polycentric mechanism). *Acta Ortopédica Mexicana, Vol. 22, No. 4*, pp. 247-253.

[14] Campos Padilla, I. Design of polycentric mechanism for knee prosthesis. Masters thesis (not published). México: National Polytechnic Institute, Advance School of Mechanical and Electrical Engineering; 2008.

[15] Xie, H., Liang, Z., Li, F. & Guo, L. (2010). The knee joint design and control of above-knee intelligent bionic leg based on magneto-rheological damper. *International Journal of Automation and Computing, Vol. 7, No. 3*, pp. 277-282.

[16] Albornoz, B. Mechanical design of virtual prototype of a transfemoral prosthetic leg that simulates natural movement of human leg. Bachelor thesis (not published). Mérida-Venezuela: Universidad de Los Andes; 2011.

[17] Lugo González, E. Design of mechanisms using genetic algorithms with application on lower limb prosthesis. Doctoral thesis. (not published). México: National Polytechnic Institute, Advance School of Mechanical and Electrical Engineering; 2010.

[18] Amador, B. T., Torrealba, R. R. & Müller-Karger, C. M. (2012). Manipulación de algoritmo genético para la obtención de dimensiones óptimas de mecanismo de cuatro barras para prótesis de rodilla (Manipulation of genetic algorithm for optimal sizing of 4-bar mechanism for knee prosthesis). Proceedings of the IV Congreso Venezolano de Bioingeniería BIOVEN'2012, San Cristóbal-Venezuela, pp. 59-62.

[19] Amador, B. T., Torrealba, R. R. & Müller-Karger C. M. (2011). Diseño conceptual de una prótesis policéntrica de rodilla para amputados transfemorales en Venezuela (Conceptual design of polycentric knee prosthesis for transfemoral amputees in Venezuela). Proceedings of the Pan American Health Care Exchanges Conference PAHCE'2011, Rio de Janeiro-Brazil, pp. 260-265.

[20] CORTEX 1.1. User's Manual. Motion Analysis; 2008.

[21] Whittle, M. W. Gait analysis an introduction. 4th Edition. Butterworth Heinemann Elsevier; 2007.

[22] Hobson, D. A. & Torfason, L. E. (1975). Computer optimization of polycentric prosthetic knee mechanisms. *Bulletin of Prosthetics Research,* pp. 187-201.

[23] Norton, R. Diseño de maquinaria: síntesis y análisis de máquinas y mecanismos. 3rd Edition. México: McGraw-Hill; 2005.

[24] Radcliffe, C. W. (2003). Biomechanics of knee stability control with four-bar prosthetic knees. ISPO Australia Annual Meeting.

[25] Amador, B., Torrealba, R., Rojas, M., Cappelletto, J. & Müller-Karger, C.M. (2012). Metodología para dimensionamiento de mecanismo policéntrico de rodilla utilizando análisis de marcha y algoritmos genéticos (Methodology to gauge a four-bar linkage prosthetic knee mechanism based on gait analysis and genetic algorithms). *Revista Ingeniería Biomédica, Vol. 6, No. 11,* pp. 30-45.

[26] Otto Bock Ibérica (2011). Rodillas [online]. Available from: http://www.ottobock.es /cps/rde/xchg/ob_es_es/hs.xsl/1943.html. (accessed February 24, 2011).

[27] Mott, R. (2006). Diseño de elementos de máquinas. 4th Edition. México: Pearson Educación.

[28] Zarrugh, M. Y. & Radcliffe, C. W. (1976). Simulation of swing phase dynamics in above-knee prostheses. *Journal of Biomechanics, Vol. 9*, pp. 283-292.

[29] Benavides, C. & Torres, A. Análisis de biomecánica digital en marcha protésica de paciente con amputación por encima de rodilla. *NOVA Publicación en Ciencias Biomédicas, Vol. 7, No. 11*, pp. 113-118. Bogotá-Colombia; 2009.

[30] Sánchez, J., Prat, J., Hoyos, J., Viosca, E., Soler, C., Comín, M., Lafuente, R., Cortés, A. & Vera, P. Biomecánica de la marcha humana normal y patológica. Valencia-España: Instituto de Biomecánica de Valencia; 2005.

[31] Farahmand, F., Rezaeian, T., Narimani, R. & Hejazi, P. (2006). Kinematic and dynamic analysis of the gait cycle of above-knee amputees. *Scientia Iranica, Vol. 13, No. 3*, pp. 261-271.

In: New Developments in Knee Prosthesis Research
Editor: Janice Stewart
ISBN: 978-1-63482-700-3

Chapter 3

Complex Procedure for Evaluating and Predicting the Wear of a Total Knee Prosthesis Tibial Tray

***Lucian Capitanu*[1], *Virgil Florescu*[2], *Liliana-Laura Badita*[3]*, *Luige Vladareanu*[1] and *Constantin Tiganesteanu*[1]**

[1]Institute of Solid Mechanics of Romanian Academy, Bucharest, Romania
[2]Technical University of Civil Engineering Bucharest, Romania
[3]National Institute for Research and Development in Mechatronics and Measurement Technique, Bucharest, Romania

Abstract

The total knee prosthesis (TKP) must allow complex movements in a cyclic charge regime: flexion-extension (FE), antero-posterior translation (APT) and internal-external rotation (IER). Still, its major drawback is failure of a tibial insert due to the subsurface cracking and delamination wear.

This chapter presents the main results of a project whose main focus was to evaluate the tibial inserts wear and to obtain the possibility to control the TKPs wear process. First, some retrieved TKPs were analysed revealing the loss of functionality, because the polyethylene tibial insert was dislocated. Next, theoretical wear studies were performed on tibial tray, based on FEM modelling, and practical studies on ball/flat couple. By applying FE and APT movements under constant compressive loading, the results showed that the fracture of tibial tray was preponderantly caused by the adhesive wear and material fatigue.

A thorough analysis was conducted with focus on phenomenon evolution, from adhesive wear pitting followed by delamination and even breaking of the insert. The failure mechanism proved being a combination of the high level of loading during normal activities and a non-

* Corresponding author e-mail: badita_l@yahoo.com

conforming contact between the femoral condyles and tibial insert. The question that arises is: Could be this phenomenon evaluated quantitatively a priori?

In order to determine the occurrence of wear in high risk areas, a predictive method was used by combining the Finite Element Analyses of contact mechanism and transfer of load in articulation, with a summation technique based on damage score estimation. Finite element simulations were performed to dynamically determine the contact area, and the contact pressure resulting in normal walking, stairs ascending and stairs descending. The finite element model used a modern contact mechanism, including friction between the metallic femoral condyles and the tibial polyethylene insert.

Summation was adopted in order to consider the cumulative effect of all activities, based on their frequency and the magnitude of the determined damage function. The computed surface of cumulative maximum damage that traverse the layers of the polyethylene insert could be identified as the cracking surface. The conclusion was that a partial answer to the question stated before could be achieved by the presented method, which was able to determine the path of the subsequent failure of the polyethylene inserts.

Based on these results, it was established the basis for implementing control strategies for a Knee Prosthesis Simulator (KPS), by Programmable Logical Controllers in Open Architecture structure. This complex procedure allowed transferring real loads from the patient artificial knee to the KPS control system, through kinematic acquisition, evaluation of joint loadings and dynamic simulation of joint contact. Practically, the data resulting from motion analysis of the patient activities would be processed by a specialized code which would determine the motion dynamic loadings of the joint. Based on data, a detailed joint tribological model would allow contact dynamics determination and generate the customized evolution of each of the controlled KPS degrees of freedoms. The use of this method would improve the accuracy of lifetime predictions, based on the experimental data obtained in a KPS.

Keywords: total knee prosthesis, wear, experimental methods, simulator

1. Introduction

Human locomotion is a natural process that is mechanically based on the relative movement between rigid levers – the skeletal bones – as the result of the movement of passive and active effectors – the muscles. Relative motion is allowed by the joints, which also play an important role in transferring the load from one bone segment to another. The load is transferred by a contact-based mechanism that involves friction and wear. Replacement of a natural joint with an artificial one affects the load transfer mechanism, and the components of the prosthesis need to allow the relative movements representing the entire range of human activity over a long period. If certain activities are prohibited or severely limited, the level of patient satisfaction will be low.

The field of prosthetic design has been strongly influenced by the low demand. If a patient has no complaints related to the functionality of the prosthesis after rehabilitation, the attention will be focused on problems related to slower-acting phenomena, such as wear, that limit the durability and lifetime of the prosthesis. Previous studies have been focused on two main areas: estimation of the load transfer mechanism in relation to the frictional contact parameters, and prediction of the wear based on the influence of those parameters on the phenomenon itself.

The knee joint is one of the most complex joints in the human body. The problem of the shape of bones and the position of ligaments, with given properties, represents the key for evaluation of knee joint properties, and also for study the knee motion. Usually, the tibial plateau and the femoral condyles are modelled by geometric approximations of the bones or by finite element descriptions obtained by computer tomography and magnetic resonance tomography [1]. Also, the points of attachment to the bones simulate the ligaments by using the spring-damper elements between the thigh and the shank [2]. Zheng et al. describe an analytical model for ligaments, muscles and contact forces between bones and menisci to examine the joint forces during exercise and restricted to the sagittal plane. Other works model the passive joint motion without load, by using five constraints in terms of three ligaments and the medial and lateral compartment of the knee to model the passive joint movement without load [3,4]. On the other hand, the surface errors can generate large errors in kinetic and kinematic simulations of articular joint contacts. To avoid such errors, the bone surfaces have to be modelled as highly curved surfaces, with unknown parameters which can be determined from experimental data.

The knee joint surface modelling must verify the geometric and also, the natural compatibility conditions. The geometric compatibility condition assures that the distance between the contact points on the two surfaces is zero, such that the penetration is avoided. The natural compatibility condition assures that normals to the surfaces at the point of contact are collinear. A method based on 2D polynomials to fit bone surface geometry is described in references [5,6,7,8]. Generally, it is observed that small errors can create penetration of the two objects in contact and result in multiple contact points.

Another method which uses polygons to represent bone surfaces is presented in reference [9]. In this paper, the natural compatibility condition is not necessarily satisfied, and the coplanar, colinearity of normals at the contact point are not verified. Using the cubic splines in investigation of parametric surface patches is investigated in [10,11,12,13,14,15], and [16]. Here, errors are possible for points at other locations on a patch which can lead to discontinuous contact points in simulations of joint contact. The use of B-splines to create geometric models of articular surfaces improve the accuracy of this extrapolation grid, but it may not represent highly curved surfaces and it requires that the digitized anatomy be regularly distributed [17]. The important parts of the knee include the end of the femur, the top of the tibia, articular cartilage (AC), meniscus cartilage, four ligaments – the anterior cruciate ligament (ACL), the posterior cruciate ligament (PCL), the medial collateral ligament (MCL), the lateral collateral ligament (LCL) – and two tendons: the quadriceps tendon (QT) and the patellar tendon (PTL) (Figure 1). The apparent space between the bones is actually occupied by articular cartilage (AC).

The articular surfaces are the large curved condyles of the femur, the flattened condyles of the tibia, and the facets of the patella. The articular cartilages (AC) act bearing surfaces and the meniscus as mobile bearings. There are large muscles in the front of the thigh (the quadriceps muscles QM) that straighten the knee (extension). The large muscles in the back of the thigh (the hamstrings) bend the knee (flexion).

The patella functions as an important lever for the quadriceps muscles, making the muscle more efficient. When bending and straightening the knee, the surfaces of the tibia and femur roll and slide on each other and the patella moves up and down against the front of the femur. The quadriceps tendon (QT) and the patellar tendon (PTL) surround the patella and help its mechanical motion and also function as a cap for the condyles of the femur.

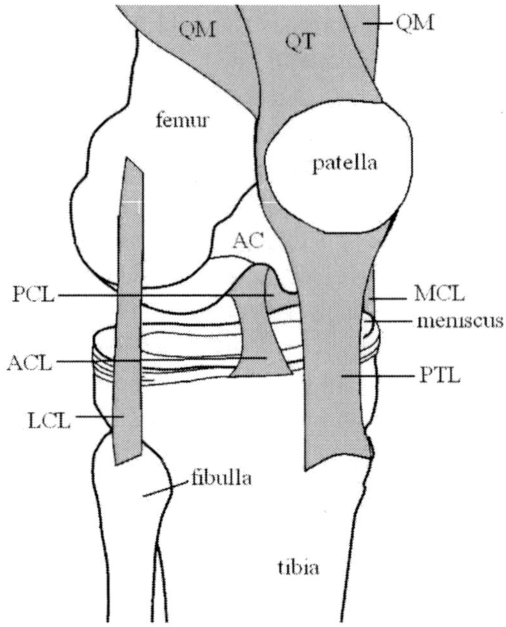

Figure 1. Schematic of the knee muscles and ligaments.

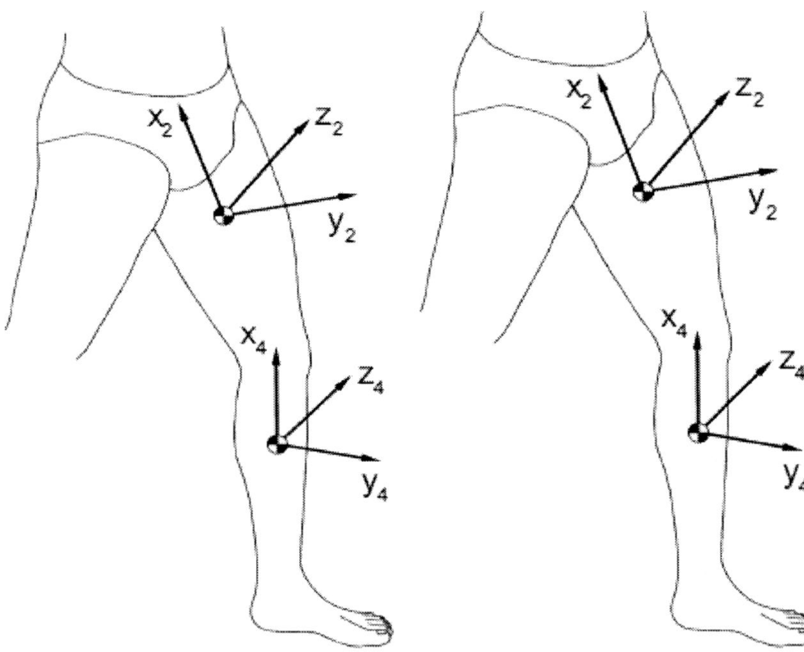

Figure 2. The axis of rotation for the left knee. The proximal and distal reference frames are shown on the left, while the axis highlighted on the right. There are three separate ranges of motion: flexion and extension (FE) take place around the medio-lateral axis of the left thigh (z_2), internal and external rotation (IER) take place around the longitudinal axis of the left calf (x_4) and abduction and adduction (AA) take place around an axis that is perpendicular to both z_2 and x_4. These three axis do not form a right-handed triad, because z_2 and x_4 are not necessarily at right angles to one another.

From kinematic point of view, the knee joint must allow the following movements:

- flexion and extension - FE (plus dorsiflexion and plantar flexion) take place around the medio-lateral axis of the proximal segment (i.e., txe axis z);
- internal and external rotation (IER) take place around the longitudinal axis of the segment (i.e., txe axis x);
- abduction and adduction (AA) take place around a floating axis that is at right angles to both the flexion / extension and internal / external rotation axis.

These angle definitions can be a little more easily understood by referring to Figure 2, which illustrates the left knee.

The forces that act upon the left knee are presented in Figure 3.

Several loading regimes are considered as characterised in [18]. For every regime, a dynamic finite element simulation of the dry-friction contact was performed to establish the contact traces and the contact pressure distribution. Those characteristics, combined with the frequencies of the activities considered (as determined in [19]), are used as the input data for a statistical evaluation of the joint loading over some period.

Previous tribological studies showed strong correlations between the contact pressure and the wear rate [20,21]. This means that different activities will lead to different levels of wear. Furthermore, for the same activity, the contact pressure will vary during the different stances of the activity [22]. Therefore, the wear phenomenon will be not a constant rate phenomenon for a given activity or between activities. The issue is even further complicated considering that different activities have different frequencies.

Further investigation is needed to understand how to quantify a priori the characteristics measures of the wear phenomenon across activities. In this study, we sought to develop a reliable method to predict the volumetric wear rate in total hip prostheses. This method involves finite element analyses (FEA) of the contact mechanism (to estimate the contact pressure variation during activity), evaluation of specific quantities that have been introduced to allow comparison between the stances within an activity and between different activities and a special summation technique that accounts for the frequency and load magnitude of every activity.

Recent clinical studies [23,24] have identified the considerable wear of the polyethylene tibial insert due to the mechanics of non-conforming contact as the main cause of prosthetic failure. In [25], Knight et al. reported that from 209 cases of primary total knee prostheses (TKP), 18 prostheses failed, with all of the tibial inserts showing wear pits and delamination. The average time to failure was approximately 80 months, close to that reported by Heck et al. in [26] (i.e., 72 months), but other studies [27,28,29,30] have shown that gross delamination could occur even earlier.

Examining an early retrieved prosthesis, Ries et al. [31] noticed gross wear pits and delamination of the tibial insert accompanied by an increase in the percentage of crystallinity at a plane coincident with the plane of delamination and the presence of a subsurface oxidation peak typically observed in ultra-high molecular weight polyethylene (UHMWPE inserts) that have been γ – irradiated in air and aged. Although the issue remains controversial, the idea that increasing the thickness of the tibial inserts would reduce wear was shown to be false. Indeed, it is the incongruence of the contact surfaces that leads to high contact pressure localised over small areas and subsequently to the fatigue wear and delamination of a polyethylene part [25, 26]. In an analysis of two retrieved TKPs (after 21 and 16 years from implantation), Oonishi et al. [32] noticed the presence of parallel scratches (oriented antero-posterior) on the femoral component and considerable delamination of the polyethylene tibial insert.

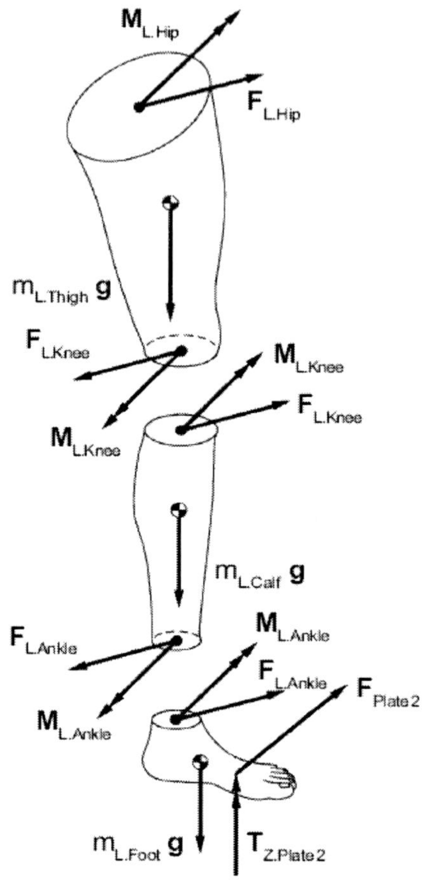

Figure 3. Free body diagrams for left foot, calf and thigh, showing the external forces acting on each segment. The forces and moments at the ankle and knee joints are equal in magnitude but opposite in direction, depending on the segment concerned (Newton's third law of motion).

2. Methodology

In our previous study [20], which is based on examination of components of retrieved prostheses, we found scratching on femoral condyles and deformations of the UHMWPE tibial insert (see Figure 4 and Figure 5).

In another study [22] were also identified characteristic marks (pits) of the fatigue wear phenomena. The insert shown in Figure 6a is from an early retrieved tibial part (the revision was performed due to the loosening of the implant).

It is possible to observe the wear pits of the contact surface, which are specific to adhesive and fatigue wear, as well as the delamination of the peripheral area of the medial part, which is an effect of fatigue wear. The tibial insert made of UHMWPE suffered and a considerable plastic deformation. Shooting of tibial insert made of polyethylene was possible by applying the touching up technique (friction of the insert with a sheet of carbon paper). In this way the insert surface was blackened, leaving visible the fatigue bites appeared on its surface due to the fatigue by cyclic mechanical strain.

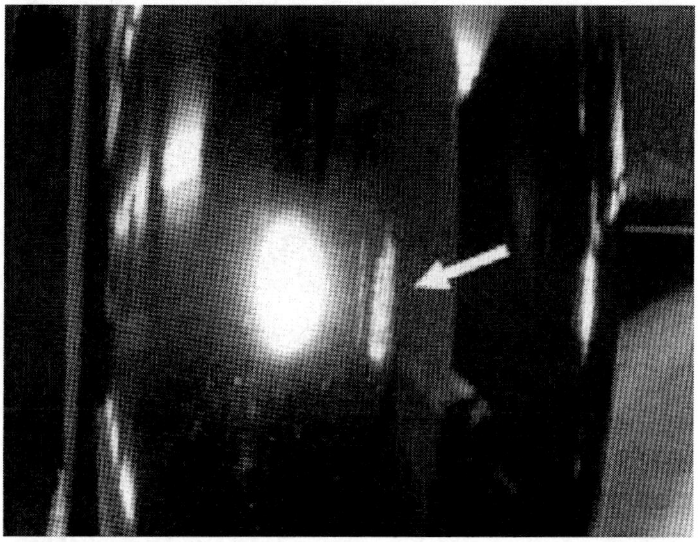

Figure 4. Image of a retrieved TKP after 21 years of operation: CoCr alloy femoral component. [32].

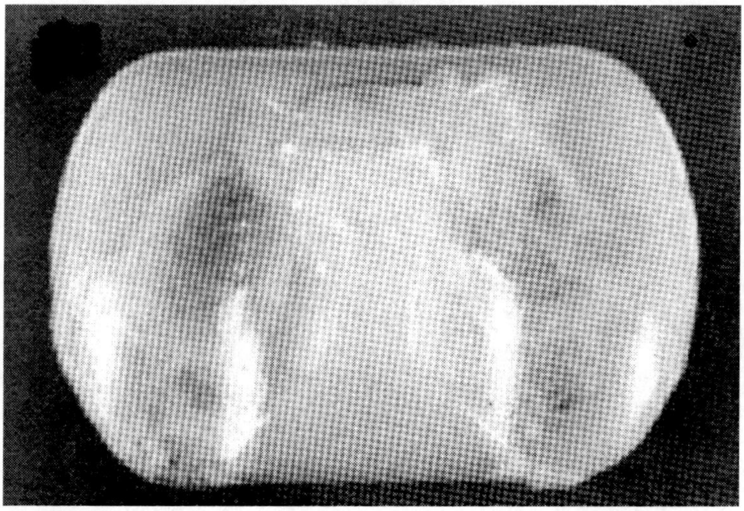

Figure 5. Optical image of a UHMWPE tibial insert retrieved after 21 years [32].

The insert shown in Figure 6b was taken from a TKP retrieved 67 months after implantation. The patient was a man of 29 years old, with weight of 115 kg, who practiced a very physically demanding sport – rugby. In this case, the fatigue wear had more catastrophic effects, including a massive loss of polyethylene in the medial part and severe delamination in the lateral part.

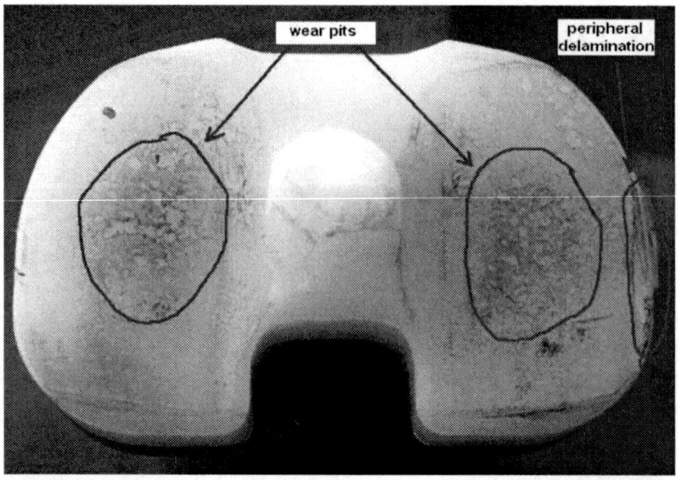

a

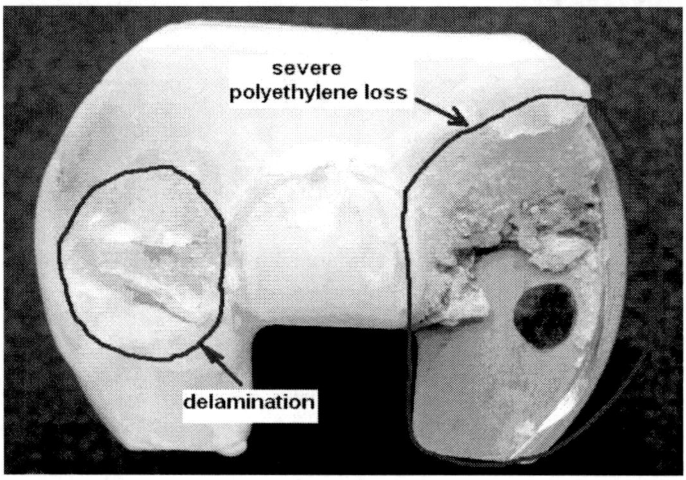

b

Figure 6. Two retrieved polyethylene inserts showing (a) fatigue pits and (b) severe delamination.

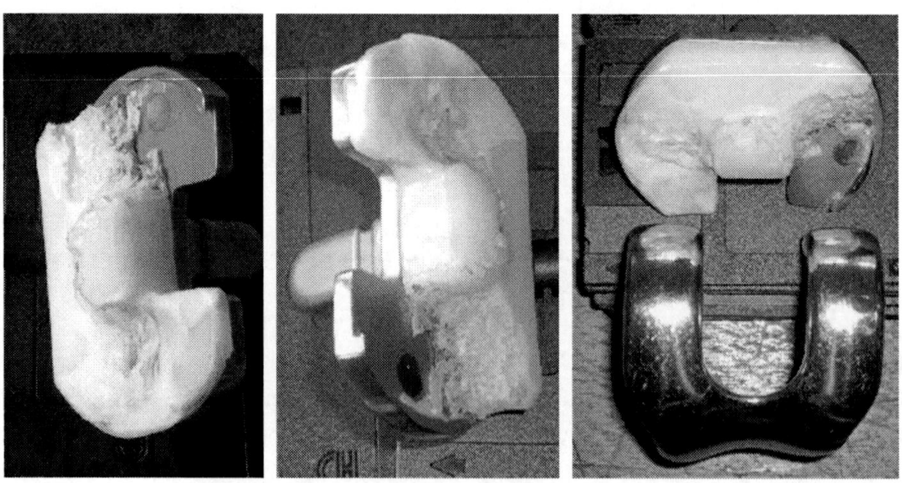

Figure 7. Pictures of the fatigue wear of the components of a total knee prosthesis.

From the qualitative evaluation of the two retrieved implants, we could conclude that the fatigue wear occurred with some wear pits at the contact surface and delamination (especially in the peripheral medial part of the tibial insert), but in time, severe damage occurred (gross delamination, massive loss of polyethylene). Due to cyclic mechanical strain and residual plastic deformation, the insert lost its fixation at the tibial plateau and was fractured. Much of the UHMWPE insert has broken away and the femoral condyle has rubbed on the metallic tibial plateau and even entered in it. This led to the need for replacement surgery of the total knee prosthesis.

To create an overview, Figure 7 presents some detailed pictures of the components of this prosthesis that we believe that represents a special case.

2.1. Mathematical Modelling of the Knee Contact Mechanism

The methodology for predicting the fatigue wear phenomena of the tibial tray combines FEA for the active loading cycles of the relevant routine activities with a summation technique that is based on computation of a cumulative estimator of damage. A finite element model of the artificial joint contact (Figure 8) was used for all analyses. The model includes one femoral condyle and one half (the medial one) of the polyethylene insert and the metallic tibial tray. For deformable parts (the tibial parts), solid brick elements with 8 nodes and 3 degrees of freedom (DOFs) per node (all three translations) are used. The femoral condyle has a toroidal shape with a radius of 22 mm in the sagittal plane (the flexion plane) and a radius of 30 mm in the transversal plane and was considered rigid. The elastic linear constitutive laws are considered for the metallic and the plastic parts. The material properties are listed in Table 1. The routine activities considered relevant for this study are the active cycles of normal walking, stair descending and stair ascending.

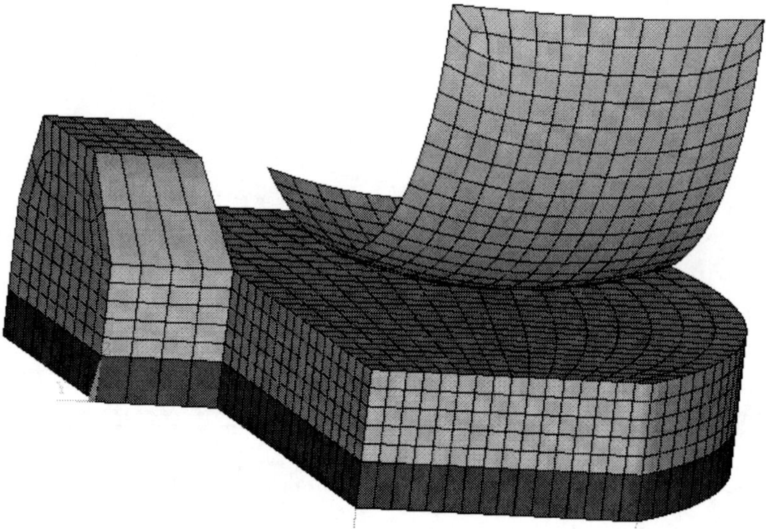

Figure 8. Finite element model used in analyses [33].

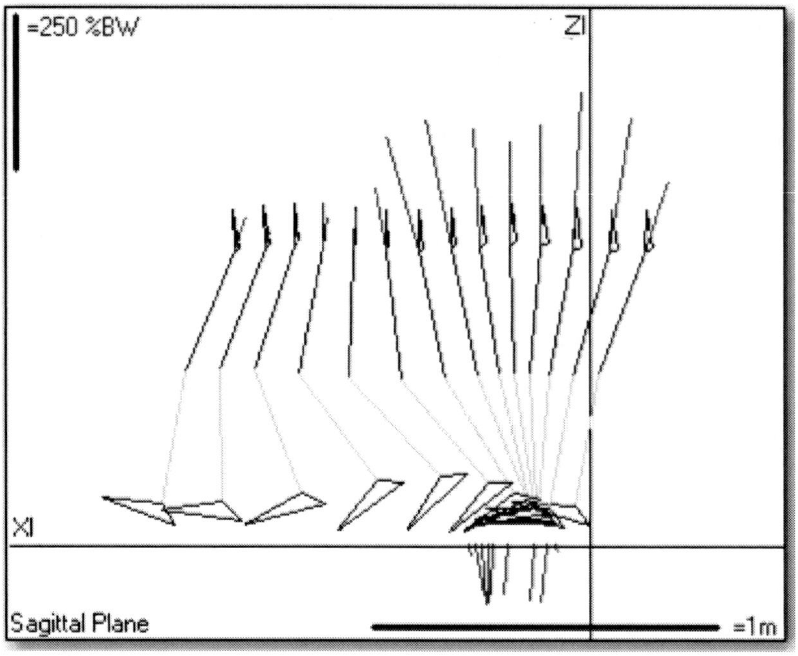

Figure 9. Kinematics of the lower member during the normal walking [18].

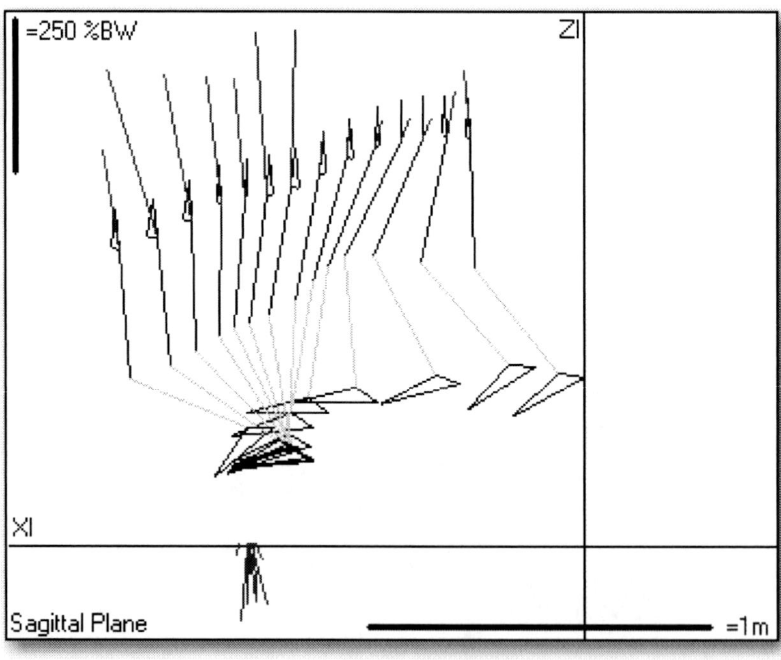

Figure 10. Kinematics of the lower member during the stair descending [18].

The kinematics of all three movements is illustrated in Figure 9, Figure 10 and Figure 11, the segmental movements of the lower member are sketched [18].

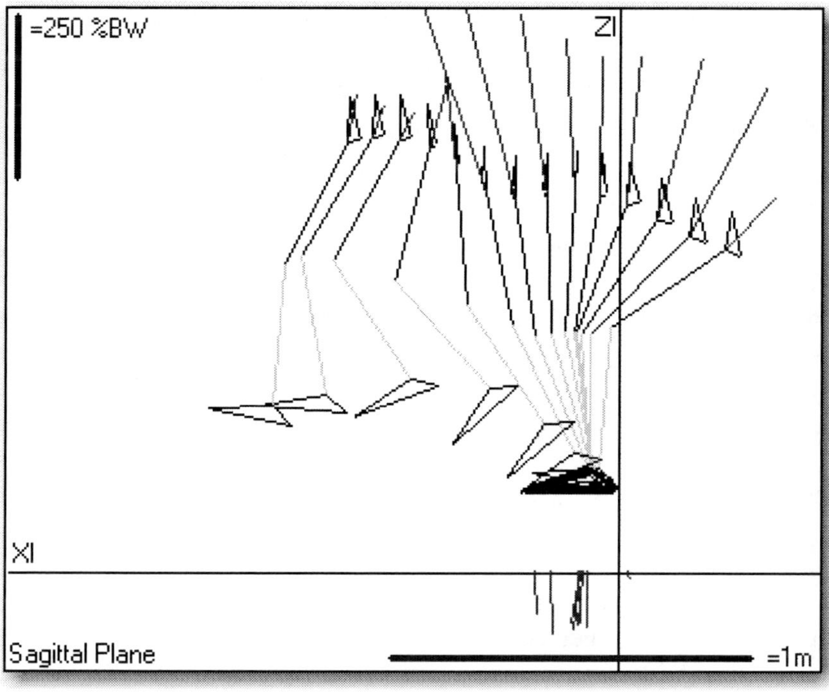

Figure 11. Kinematics of the lower member during the stair ascending [18].

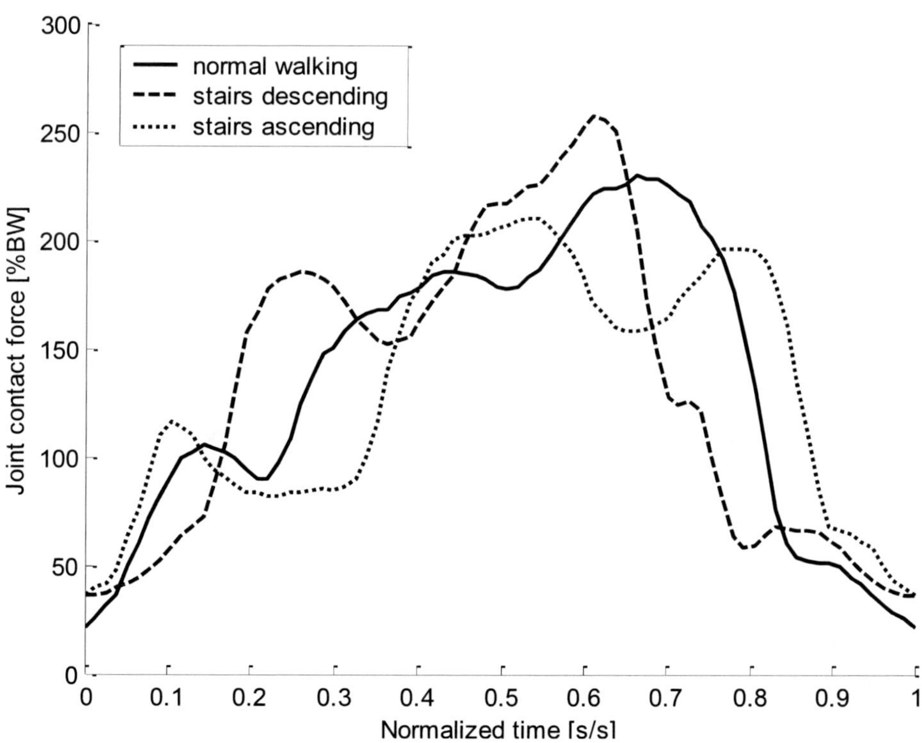

Figure 12. Loading of joint surfaces of the lower member (contact force) [35].

Table 1. The mechanical properties of the materials used in FEA

Material	Young's modulus, E (GPa)	Poisson ratio's, ν	Remarks
Co-Cr alloy	200	0.30	From ISO 5832-4
UHMWPE	1.06	0.36	From Lewis [34]

In Figure 12 the compressive forces of the contact are listed and compared for all activities considered [35].

In Figures 13 and 14, two determinants of the kinematic conditions (the flexion angle and the internal-external rotation of the tibia) are plotted [18].

Based on the model of the artificial knee joint contact presented in Figure 8, the compressive force is applied to the tibial tray (as the distributed pressure on the lower basis of it).

The two rotations (flexion and internal-external rotation) dynamically constrain the femoral part. We considered that the actual level of flexion (not higher than 70 degrees) does not induce an antero-posterior translation (which usually appears when the ligaments are overstrained), as it does for extended flexion.

The contact mechanism includes rolling and sliding of the two joint surfaces – the femoral condylar toroidal surface and the planar surface of the tibial insert; the friction obeys Coulomb's law with a constant friction coefficient of 0.12 [36].

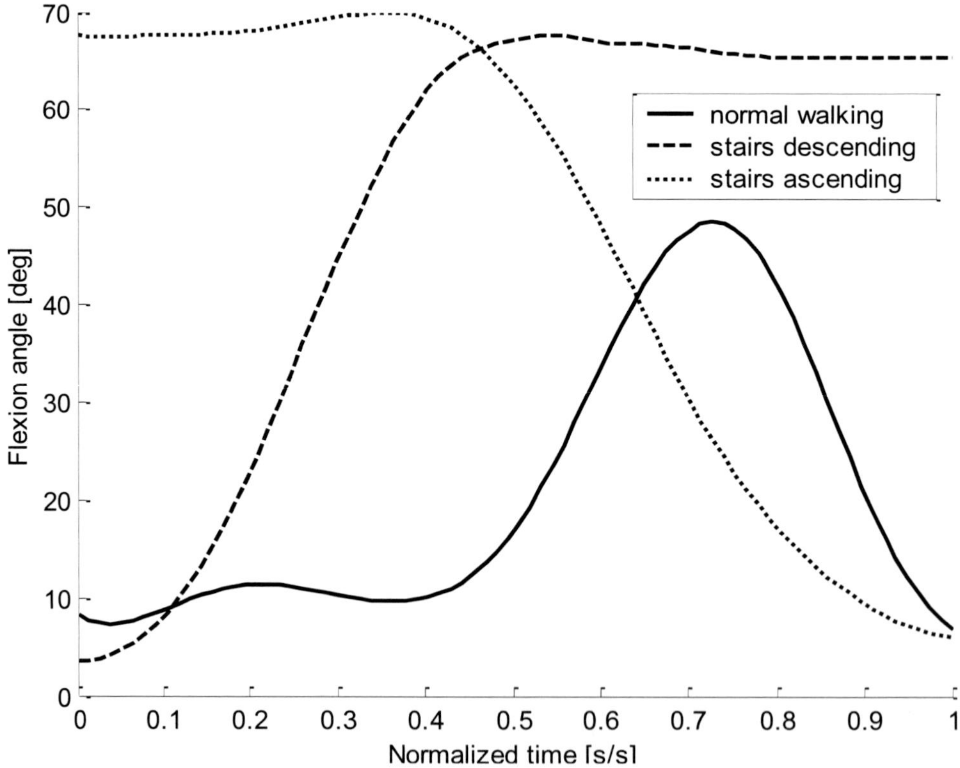

Figure 13. Kinematics of joint surfaces of the lower member (flexion angle) [18].

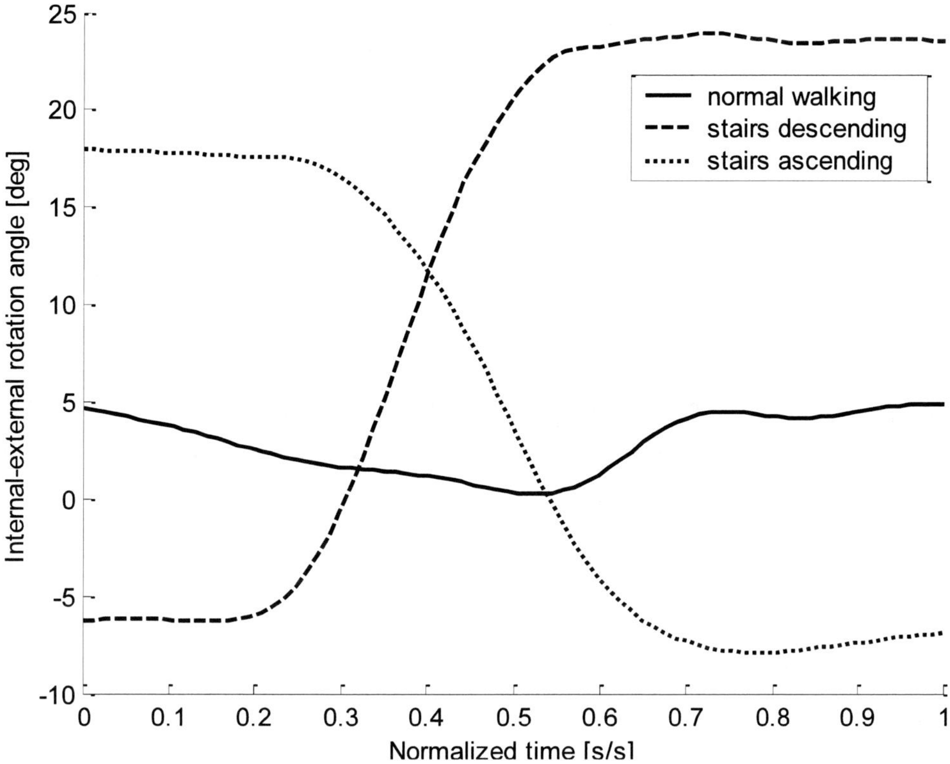

Figure 14. Kinematics of joint surfaces of the lower member (internal-external rotation angle) [18].

For every activity, a damage estimator can be computed from the variation of the shear maximum principal stress in every element [37].

$$D_f^k = \sum_{i=1}^{n} \frac{1}{2} \left| \tau_{i+1} - \tau_i \right| \cdot \left(\left| \tau_{i+1} \right| + \left| \tau_i \right| \right) \tag{1}$$

where: D_f^k - damage function for activity k and

τ_i - shear maximum stress on elements for time t_i

The effect of all activities could be cumulated by evaluating a weighted sum:

$$D_f^{tot} = \sum w_k D_f^k \tag{2}$$

where the weights are depending on the frequency of the activity.

To validate our assumption of a rigid-to-flexible contact, we estimated the contact stiffness of the two continua that are contact with each other by the following formula:

$$\gamma = \frac{E}{4 \cdot \left(1 - \nu^2\right)}. \tag{3}$$

Using formula (3), one could obtain the ratio of the stiffness of the two continua, which is large enough to support our assumption:

$$\frac{\gamma_{fin.codyle}}{\gamma_{UHMWPE}} \approx 200.$$

In our analysis, we obtained the dynamic distribution of the pressure, which means that we determined the value of the contact pressure for every point on the surface and in every moment. If we denote the contact surface with S and the duration of the active cycle of a specific activity with T, we can determine the contact pressure as a function of time and position:

$$p(t,x); t \in [0,T], x \in S$$

One could define the instantaneous maximum pressure as:

$$p_m(t) = \max\{p(t,x); x \in S\}$$

and the maximum pressure as:

$$p_M = \max\{p(t,x); x \in S, t \in [0,T]\}$$

These two measures are specific for the level of the loading at a specific moment of the activity or for the entire period. Based on the functions defined above, we can evaluate the relative measure of the proximity to the maximum area of pressure, designated as the "instantaneous index of pressure":

$$\tilde{p}(t;x) = \frac{p(t,x)}{p_m(t)} \tag{4}$$

For every moment of time, we can determine the level of loading by:

$$\lambda(t) = \frac{p_m(t)}{p_M} \tag{5}$$

The volume of the material removed by wear is:

$$V = kPnL = \int_0^T k(t)P(t)vdt \tag{6}$$

where

$$v = const. = \frac{L}{T} \tag{7}$$

is the velocity of the relative movement of the frictional couple (assumed constant here), and $P(t)$ is the result of contact determined by integrating the contact pressure over the entire interface surface:

$$P(t) = \int_S p(t,x)\,dA \tag{8}$$

As mentioned above, experimental tests showed some correlation between the contact pressure and the wear rate. By testing the CoCr/UHMWPE hip prostheses in a hip joint simulator, Wang et al. [21] found that the wear factor could be expressed as:

$$k = C\sigma_0^n \tag{9}$$

They also established the values for the constant C and the exponent n:

$$C = 7.99 \cdot 10^{-6} \qquad n = -0.653$$

By substituting (7), (8) and (9) in (6), we can obtain the volume of the material removed during a single activity:

$$V = nC\frac{L}{T}p_M^{n+1} \cdot \int_0^T\int_S \left(\frac{p_m(t)}{p_M}\right)^{n+1}\left(\frac{p(x,t)}{p_m(t)}\right)dAdt = \\ nC_M^{n+1}L\int_S \frac{1}{T}\int_0^T \lambda^{n+1} \cdot \tilde{p}(t,x)dtdA \tag{10}$$

For more than one activity, we can perform an algebraic summation as follows:

$$V_{med} = \sum_i V_i = \sum_i \left(n_i C p_M^{n+1} L \int_S \frac{1}{T}\int_0^T \lambda^{n+1} \cdot \tilde{p}(t,x)dtdA \right) = \\ \int_S \left(\sum n_i C p_M^{n+1} L \cdot \frac{1}{T}\int_0^T \lambda^{n+1} \cdot \tilde{p}(t,x)dt \right) dA \tag{11}$$

One can see that the integrated

$$I = \sum_i n_i Cp_M^{n+1} L \cdot \frac{1}{T} \int_0^T \lambda^{n+1} \cdot \widetilde{p}(t,x) dt \qquad (12)$$

is a function of position only, and it may be a good measure of the tendency of some areas of the contact interface to be affected by wear.

This means that a map of the distribution of the values of this integrated could be a good predictor for the geometrical features on the joint surfaces. We have denoted this integrated (either summed over activities or specific for every activity) as being a wear geometrical descriptor.

Performing the dynamic analyses of the contact between the femoral metallic condyles and the polyethylene tibial insert (in the conditions described above), it is possible to determine the characteristics of the contact mechanism in the artificial knee (Figure 15).

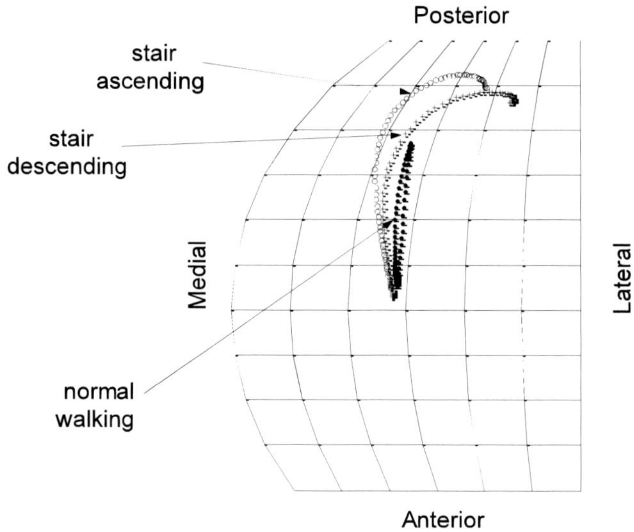

Figure 15. The contact paths for all three cases considered.

For example, the trajectories of the contact spot for all three activities are plotted on a sketch of the medial part of the polyethylene insert (see Figure 15).

By examining the sketch, one can see that not all activities involve extension of the knee – this means that only the median and posterior parts of the insert are used. For normal walking, the trajectory is a closed curve (like a hysteretic loop).

The stair ascending and stair descending trajectories are quite similar (although they are opposite in direction). Both activities have a large internal-external rotation (for stair ascending, loading occurs at the beginning of the cycle; for stair descending, loading occurs at the end of it). It can be seen that the normal walking loading cycle will affect the median area of the medial part of the insert, and the stair ascending and descending activities will have their maxima located in the posterior parts of the insert.

As expected, due to the geometry of the contact (the joint surfaces are a toroidal surface for the femoral condyle and a plane surface for the tibial insert), it is clear that the contact spot will have an elliptical form with the major axis oriented transversally to the sagittal plane of the femoral condyle. The maximum contact pressure is a good estimate of the intensity of the loading. The variation in time of this contact parameter will follow the variation of the magnitude of loading (see Figure 16).

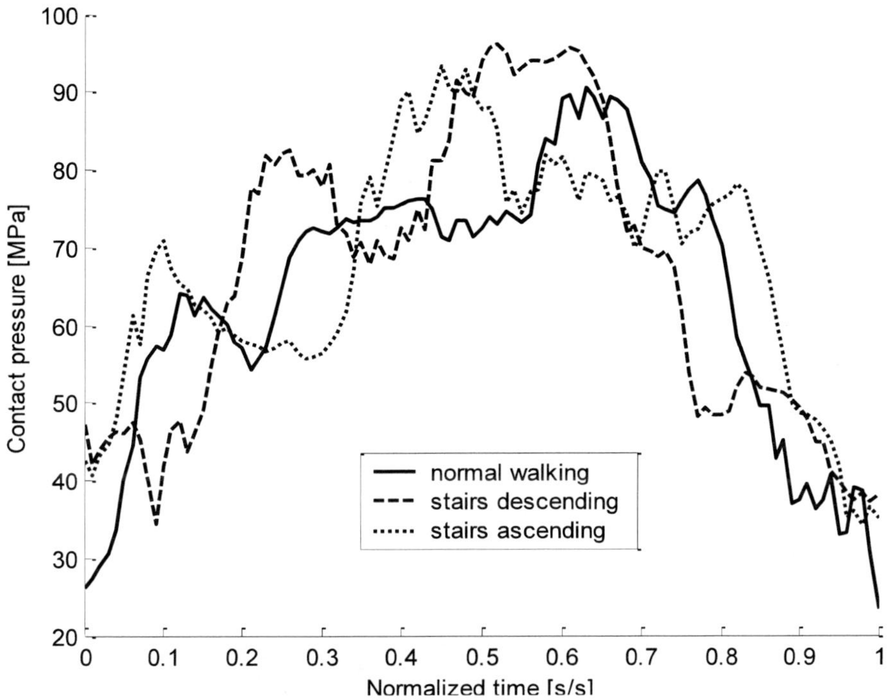

Figure 16. The contact pressure variation for all three cases considered.

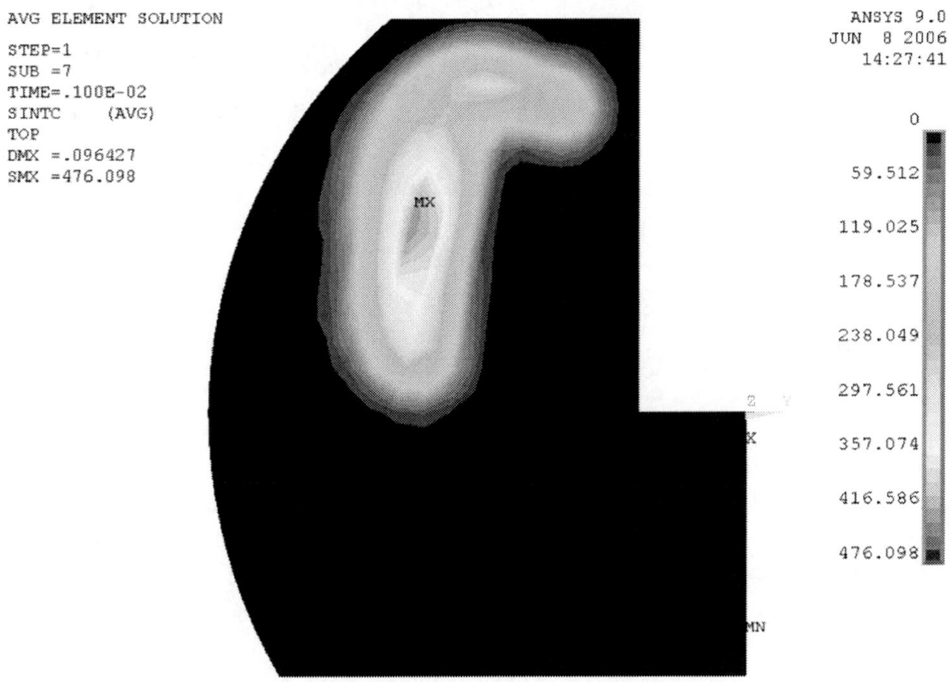

Figure 17. The damage score map at the contact surface.

An initial step maximum can be seen for all activities, corresponding to the initiation of the movement – the contact between the foot and the floor. The contact pressure is important as an estimator of the loading magnitude, but it is even more important for estimating the fatigue wear and the maximum shear stress, as the parameter used in the damage estimator, as stated by formula (1).

From the contact mechanism, which involves both rolling and frictional sliding, the maximum shear stress will be located under the contact surface at a distance dependent on the aspect ratio of the elliptical contact spot.

Using the cumulative estimator defined in formula (2), the areas where the damage is likely to occur can be identified from the cumulative distributions plotted in Figure 17 and Figure 18 (the L-shaped region in a different colour). It can be seen that the most affected areas are the medial and posterior parts of the tibial insert.

One could may also notice that the maximum damage will occur at the subsurface of the insert (where the shear stresses from normal walking is maximal), which is usually the starting plane of severe delamination.

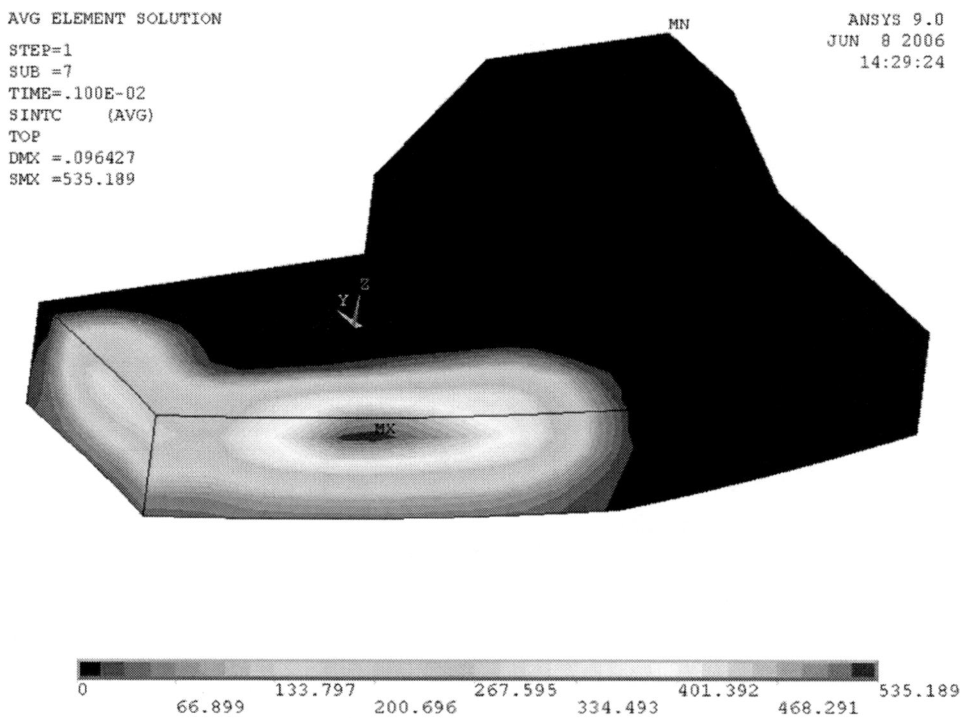

Figure 18. The damage score map in the subsurface.

The magnitudes of the damage estimator (~477 MPa^2 at the surface and ~535 MPa^2 in the subsurface) [38] are in concordance with the results of Sathasivam and Walker [37], who obtained a damage score of ~230 MPa^2 for a constant loading of 1,000 N (approx. 120% BW), representing one half of the maximum load from normal walking or from stair ascending or stair descending activities.

2.2. Experimental Modelling

By replacing the natural joint, the knee prosthesis must allow the same complex movements: flexion – extension (FE), antero-posterior translation (APT) and internal-external rotation (IER), all of them in a cyclic loading regime. Experimental modelling is devoted to the determination of the wear of a UHMWPE prosthetic tibial tray, using studies on ball/ flat couple under constant compressive loading.

Two bodies that are in contact in a point become deformed when pressed against each other, thus creating a small contact surface. Hertz has calculated the deformations and stresses in the case of homogenous, isotropic, frictionless, linear elastic bodies.

For two different materials, having the elasticity modulus E_1 and E_2, and the Poisson ratios ν_1 and ν_2, the equivalent elasticity modulus E is defined, through the relation:

$$E = \frac{E_1 E_2}{\left(1-\nu_1^2\right)E_2 + \left(1-\nu_2^2\right)E_1} \tag{13}$$

For a ball on flat couple, where the ball is made out of CoCr alloy, with the elasticity modulus $E_1 = 1.9 \cdot 10^4$ daN/mm^2, and the Poisson's coefficient $\nu_1 = 0.3$ and the plane sample made of UHMWPE ($\nu_2 = 0.36$ and $E_2 = 106$ daN/mm^2), the equivalent elasticity modulus is $E = 242$ daN/mm^2. Considering two revolution bodies having boundary surfaces with $1/R_1$ and $1/R_2$ curvatures, one introduces the relative curvature given by:

$$\frac{1}{R} = \frac{1}{R_1} + \frac{1}{R_2}. \tag{14}$$

If one of the surfaces is concave, the curvature of that surface will be considered negative.

For the particular case of the contact between a sphere of radius r and a plane, we have:

$$\frac{1}{R_1} = \frac{1}{r} \text{ and } \frac{1}{R_2} \to 0.$$

Applying a F compression load between the two parts leads to the appearance of a contact area, due to surface deformation.

The F compression force causes a h movement of the center of the sphere, through its penetration in the flat body, according to relation:

$$h = \left(\frac{9F^2}{16rE^2}\right)^{1/3}. \tag{15}$$

The relation between the circle diameter l (of the spherical contact spot) and the penetration h is:

$$l^2 = 4 \cdot r \cdot h.$$

Using (15) it result the diameter of the contact spot:

$$l = \left(\frac{6F \cdot r}{E} \right)^{1/3}. \qquad (16)$$

3. Determination of Wear Parameters

An experimental device was created for the simulation of the wear process of total knee prosthesis components. For this purpose, a ball/ flat couple was used. It consists of a ball made of CoCr alloy, simulating a condyle of the femoral component, and a UHMWPE disk placed underneath representing the tibial component. The thickness of UHMWPE disk was 5 or 10 mm and was mounted on a CoCr alloy plate. The movement made and the applied loadings were based on biomedical studies. The complex movement consisted in: flexion-extension (FE), antero-posterior translation (APT) and internal-external rotation (IER). The FE movement is applied to the ball and APT and IER to the disk (Figure 19).

These movements were made by intermediate of a rod – handle mechanism. The movements' variation in time was almost sinusoidal, a movement cycle period being of 1s. The kinematics is very similar to that used by V. Saikko, T. Ahlroos and O. Calonius at the Helsinki University of Technology [39].

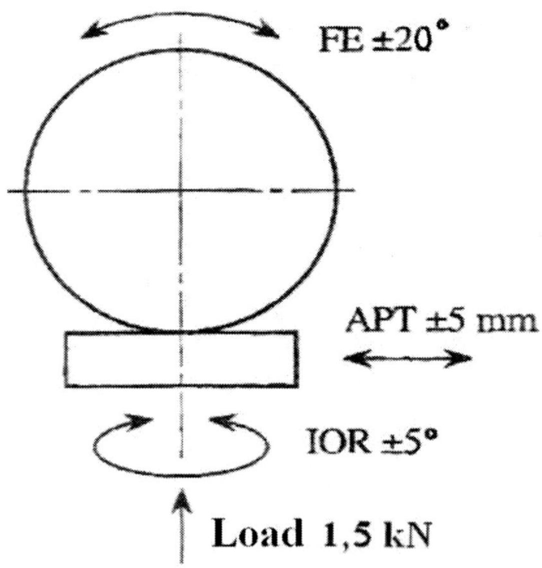

Figure 19. The friction couple kinematics.

The amplitude of the FE movement was of 40^0. For FE movement only, the sliding distance between the extreme positions would be of 20 mm, for a 54 mm diameter ball. Anyway, the APT movement with the amplitude of 10 mm, was synchronized with the FE movement so that the maximum flexion would coincide with the maximum posterior translation of the disk, and the maximum extension with the corresponding maximum anterior translation. This has shortened the sliding distance between the extreme positions. Due to both movements, the contact spot moved relatively cyclic on the disk surface.

The rod – handle mechanism was created so the phase angle between the IER and the APT sinusoidals is $\pi/2$. As a consequence, the locus of the point where the force is applied to the disk (meaning the geometrical path of a theoretical contact point) was an antisymmetric narrow figure, in the shape of eight (see Figure 20).

The parametric equations of the curve (C_1) are:

$$\begin{aligned} x_1 &= d \cdot k \cdot \cos(\varphi_0 \cdot k), \\ y_1 &= d \cdot k \cdot \sin(\varphi_0 \cdot k); \\ k &\in [0,1], \end{aligned} \tag{17}$$

where:

- k is the adimensionalized time;
- d is the relative translation between the surfaces;
- φ_0 is the maximum IER angle.

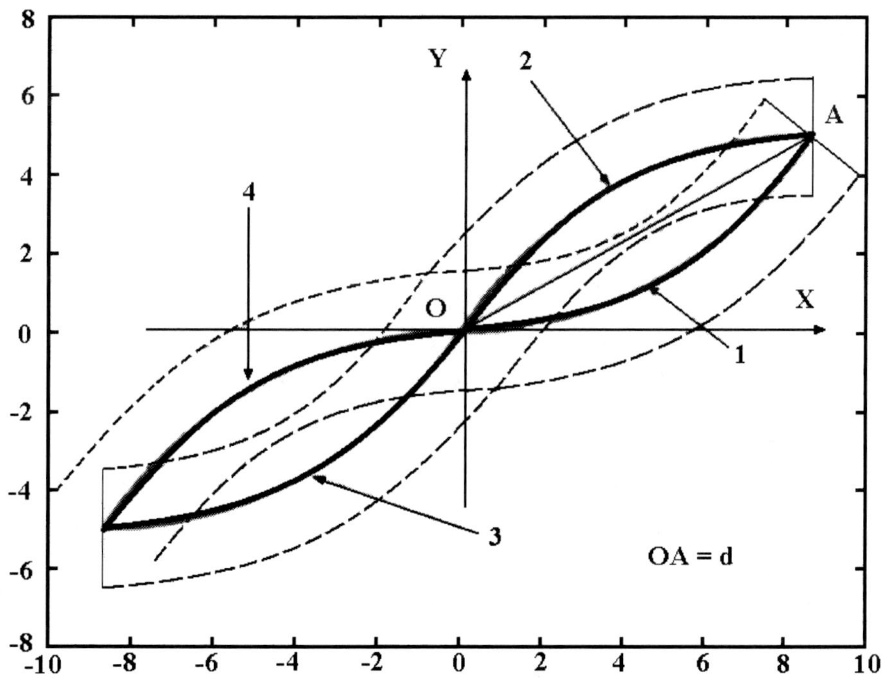

Figure 20. The trajectories of the contact point between the ball and the plane.

Similarly, the equations of curve (C_2) are:

$$x_2 = d \cdot \cos\varphi_0 - d \cdot k \cdot \cos(\varphi_0 \cdot k),$$
$$y_2 = d \cdot \sin\varphi_0 - d \cdot k \cdot \sin(\varphi_0 \cdot k);\quad (18)$$
$$k \in [0,1],$$

The curves (C_3) and (C_4) are anti-symmetrically defined:

$$x_3 = -x_1, y_3 = -y_1, k \in [0,1]\quad (19)$$

$$x_4 = -x_2, y_4 = -y_2, k \in [0,1]\quad (20)$$

The length of one of the curves is:

$$L = \int_0^1 \sqrt{\left[(x_1')^2 + (y_1')^2\right]} \cdot dk\quad (21)$$

From (17) it results:

$$L = \int_0^1 \sqrt{1+k^2} \cdot dk.\quad (22)$$

The area of the circular segment (S_w) defining the vertical profile of the wear imprint is:

$$S_w = \frac{r^2}{2} \cdot \left[\arcsin\left(\frac{l}{2r}\right) - \frac{l}{2r}\right]\quad (23)$$

where l is the width of the imprint.

The volume of the theoretical imprint can be calculated as:

$$V_w = 2S_w \cdot L.\quad (24)$$

The APT movement was realized so that lever fixed on the FE shaft led to a low – friction movement of a straight, horizontal beam, coupled to a force transducer. The transducer signal was proportional to the friction force between the ball and the disk.

This method allows determination of the friction coefficient μ.

The first experiments carried out, using only FE and APT movements, led to a very small wear rate. By adding the IER movement, the wear rate increased, the wear phenomenon becoming more complex.

The vertical loading of 1.5 kN was constant, corresponding to the maximum load induced in the knee by the routine activities. Due to translations, the stress in the disk modifies in a cyclic manner, even for a constant compression force.

The disk samples (having a diameter of 40 mm) were made out of very high density polyethylene, type Gur 1050. The tests were made on different disks. Oxidation was simulated through the ageing of the polyethylene after the gamma irradiation. The lower part of the disk was placed on a level support of CoCr alloy. The lubricant was sterilized, filtered physiological serum with a low content of proteins and endotoxins, diluted 1:1, without additives. The tests were carried out at room temperature. During the tests, the value of the friction force was also achieved.

The duration of the tests was of $5 \cdot 10^6$ cycles, at a frequency of 1 Hz. The tests were stopped every 500.000 cycles in order to change the lubricant.

The elastic deformation of the polyethylene under pressure has as a consequence an increase of its radius in the contact area. By noting r – the radius of the undeformed contact area and r_m – the radius of the deformed area by the contact, it can be seen in Figure 21 that $r_m > r$.

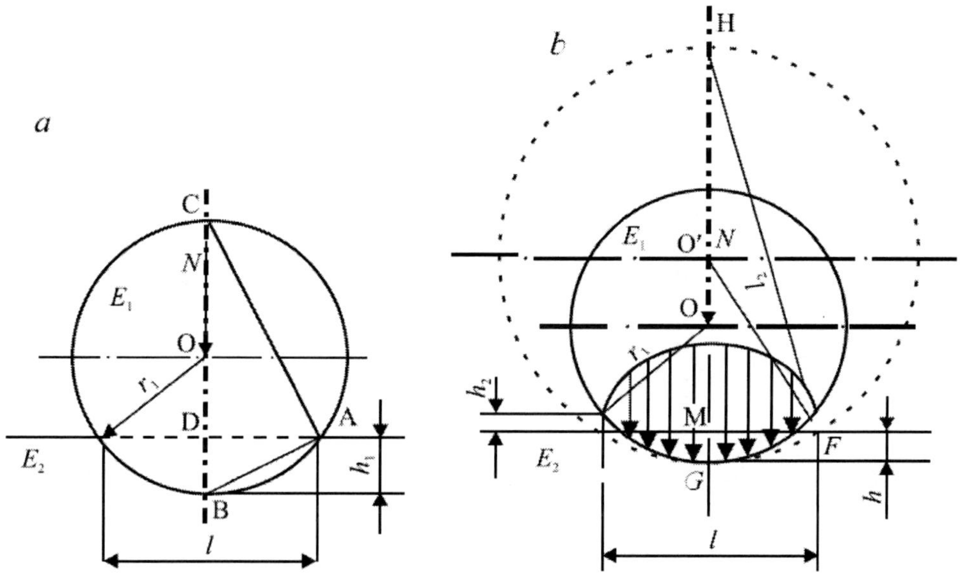

Figure 21. Elastic deformation under load of the plane component, in contact area: theoretical case (a) and (b) practical case.

The equivalent curvature radius in the point where l_m imprint width was measured can be calculated from (16):

$$r_m = \frac{E \cdot l_m^3}{6F}. \tag{25}$$

The volume of material removed through the wear from the flat element will be:

$$V_w = \frac{L_m \cdot r_m^2}{2} \cdot \left[\arcsin\left(\frac{l_m}{2r}\right) - \frac{l_m}{2r} \right] \tag{26}$$

where L_m is the measured length of the imprint.

Solving numerical, one obtains the solution:

$$R_m = 27{,}3212 \text{ mm} \approx 1{,}012r.$$

Practically, the microscopic measurement of the imprints width in five established points allows computation of the medium width of the imprint. Based on this value, the volume of worn material of the flat polyethylene element V_w is determined as well as medium depth of the layer removed through wear h_{wm}. The results obtained from the experimental trials, for a constant force of 1500 N, having a FE of ± 5 mm, are presented in Table 2.

The tests 1 and 2 were performed on polyethylene disks having a 5 mm width, and tests 3, 4 and 5 on disks having 10 mm width. The theoretical length of the friction distance covered by the contact spot, on each movement cycle, was 10 mm. The measurements carried out with the microscope have shown an effective increase of these values, probably caused by the shear stresses occurred at the edges of contact area.

Table 2. Wear of polyethylene disks and average of friction coefficient

No	Wear	Wear factor	Wear pit dimensions			μ
			L	W	D	
1	72.26	0.935	10.3	1.32	0.6	0.036
2	128.56	1.679	10.1	1.61	1.3	0.053
3	71.31	0.914	10.4	1.31	0.5	0.035
4	120.40	1.514	10.6	1.56	0.9	0.034
5	112.48	1.428	10.5	1.52	1.0	0.047

W - Wear (10^{-3} mm^3); Wear factor (10^{-11} mm^3/Nm); L – Length (mm); W – Width (mm); D – Depth (10^{-3} mm).

For tests 2 and 3, the UHMWPE samples were sterilized through γ irradiation and aged through air convection. Tests 1 and 4 were carried out the samples that were not irradiated and test 5 on samples that were irradiated but not aged.

The wear factor was determined based on Archard's relation [40]:

$$V_w = F \cdot k \cdot v \cdot t \tag{27}$$

where:

V_w – volume of material removed through wear (cm^3);
F – working load (daN);
v – relative sliding speed (cm/s);
t – test duration (h);
k – wear factor (cm^3·s/daN·m·h).

Relation (27) expresses a general law for the dependency of the wear as a function of the compressive force between the bodies in contact and the space covered by friction.

Therefore, we can write:

$$k = V_w / (F \cdot v \cdot t) = V_w / (F \cdot L_f), \tag{28}$$

where L_f is the space covered by friction.

Table 2 also shows the medium values of the friction coefficient, determined based on the measurements carried out by intermediate of the force transducer coupled on the bearing with low linear friction, part of the generator of the APT movement.

Aiming to improve the performance of the knee prosthesis simulator (KPS) control system a new method has been developed for hybrid position – force control on five DOFs in an open architecture with PC interfaced multi-processor PLC system in order to obtain new control functions. Mainly, this architecture allows for real time control, having two sources of data: measurements of the dynamic forces and of the static precision as interaction between the work piece and the environment [41, 42]. The hybrid position – force control in Cartesian coordinates, conceived as a control system in open architecture (OAH), is realized by processing in real time the Jacobean matrix obtained from direct kinematics through the Denevit – Hartenberg method with the calculus of the inverse Jacobean matrix for back loop control [43].

The studying method produced a control system for KPS on 5 DOFs which maintains a constant force of vertical pressure on the tibial component. First considered is a mathematical model determined off-line based on the studies done by the authors, from which the trajectories for femoral and tibial movement are generated online.

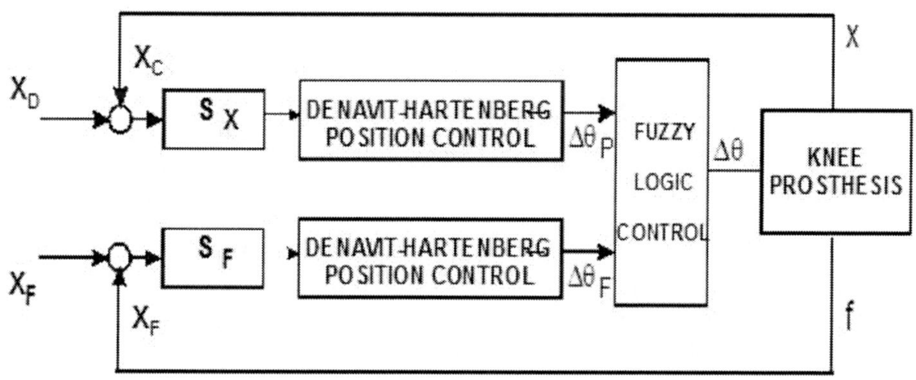

Figure 22. The general structure of hybrid control.

The trajectory of the tibial movement is controlled in real time and is composed of 4 movement functions corresponding to 4 DOFs. The femoral movement trajectory, which represents the 5-th DOF, is synchronized with the tibial movement trajectory through the freedom axis trajectory control accordingly to the mathematical model determined off-line and the chosen law of movement. The control system has 4 knee prosthesis simulator stations. Each station allows, individually or jointly with the others, the Cartesian force and torque (*Fx, Fy, Fz, Mx, My, Mz*) to be monitored continuously or at periodical intervals using load cells. Supplementary, the temperature control for 8 measurement points is available.

Hybrid position – force control of knee prosthesis equipped with compliant joints must take into consideration the passive compliance within the system [44, 45]. The generalized surface on which the knee prosthesis labours must be defined in a constrained space with 5

DOFs, with position constraints along the normal to this surface and force constraints along the tangents. On the basis of these two constraints, the general structure of hybrid position – force control is described in Figure 22, and the general constructive scheme is presented in Figure 23.

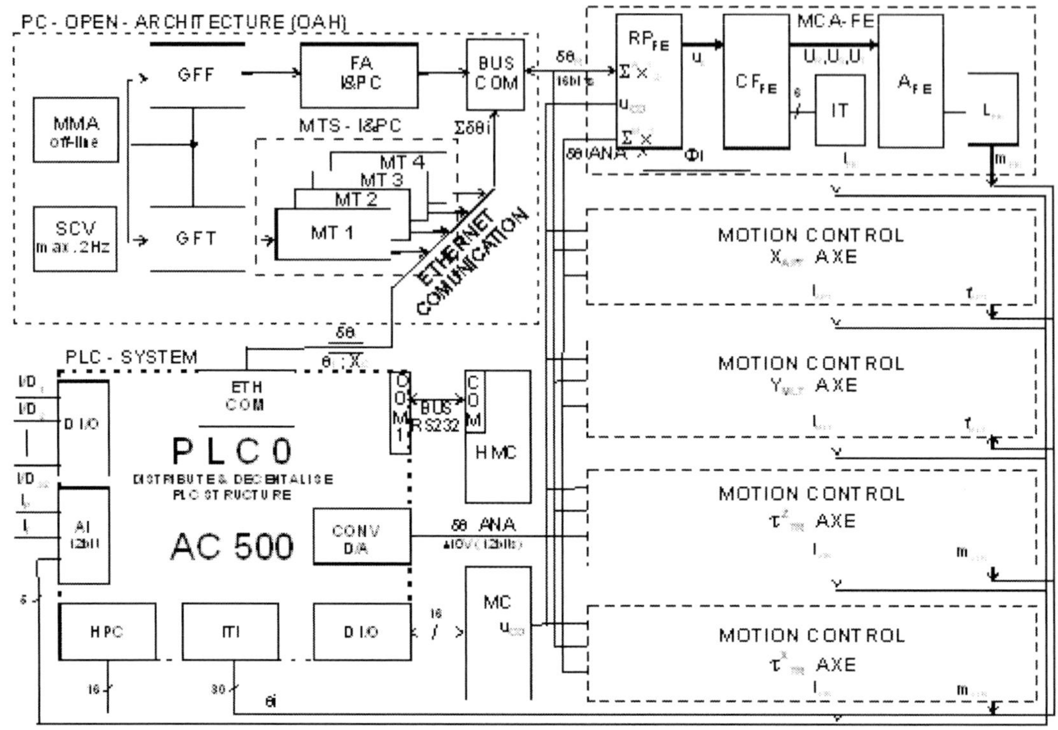

Figure 23. The general scheme for hybrid control.

Out of simplification considerations the coordinate transformations are not noted. The variables X_C and F_C represent the Cartesian position, respectively the Cartesian force exerted upon the environment. Considering X_C and F_C as expressed in environment – specific coordinates, the selection matrixes S_x and S_f can be determined, which are diagonal matrixes with 0 and 1 as diagonal elements, and fulfil the relation:

$$S_x + S_f = L_d \tag{29}$$

In more recent approaches [46], S_x and S_f are methodically deduced from the kinematical constraints imposed by the working environment. Let A and B be two full column rank matrices spanning the twist and wrench spaces of constraint. They satisfy the relation:

$$A \cdot B = 0 \tag{30}$$

Then S_x and S_f can be determined through the relations:

$$S_f = (B^t \cdot \psi^{-1} \cdot B)^{-1} \cdot B^t \cdot \psi^{-1} \tag{31}$$

$$S_x = (A^t \cdot \psi \cdot A)^{-1} \cdot A^t \cdot \psi \tag{32}$$

where Ψ is usually a symmetrical, positive-definite matrix.

It is easily verifiable that [42,44,46] using any of the above approaches, S_x and S_f always fulfil:

$$rang(S_x) + rang(S_f) = 6;\; S_x^t \cdot S_f = 0 \tag{33}$$

The control rules are design to bring to zero the position errors $e_x = \Delta\theta_P$ and force errors $e_f = \Delta\theta_F$.For an ideal control system, the behaviour of knee prosthesis is defined by:

$$S_x \cdot (v_{des} - v) = 0 \tag{34}$$

$$S_f \cdot (f_{des} - f) = 0 \tag{35}$$

where v is the velocity, f is the force and the index "*des*" specifies the reference parameter (the desired value). Velocity constraint is the only one taken into consideration here and constraint position is satisfied as a consequence.

The relations (34) and (35) lead to the following conclusion: with the aid of hybrid control, the knee prosthesis acts as a rigid body, without mass, submitted to an external force f_{des} and connected through an ideal kinematic constraint to another body, whose velocity is v_{des}.

A reference position interpolation for 4 tibial axes is provided through multi-tasking system. The experimental results are in good agreement with the theoretical predicted results for trajectory control, showing the possibility of practical implementation of control strategies for the KPS by using PLCs (Programmable Logical Controller). The monitored parameters are available for evaluating the prosthesis materials, implant wear, change of the friction rate, tribology behaviour, etc. The developed method is also useful for the validation of the analytical models which are to be further developed to portray the dynamic behaviour and timeline behaviour of the knee prosthesis.

For patients operated for TKR, dynamic characteristics calculated based on the estimator from Eq. 1 change compared to the normal patients, as shown in Figure 24, Figure 25 and Figure 26.

A significant difference between the clinical cases and the normal people is clearly observed.

Performing the dynamic analyses of the contact between the femoral metallic condyles and the polyethylene tibial insert (in the conditions described above) one could determinate the characteristics of the contact mechanism in the artificial knee.

Examining the graphs plotted in Figure 4, one could see that if for normal gait there is no extension – i.e., only the median and posterior parts of insert are used, for cerebral palsy gait some extension occurs (up to 10 degrees) and the anterior part of the insert will be also loaded.

A quantitative analysis of the curves plotted in Figure 24, Figure 25 and Figure 26 shows that for cerebral palsy gait, the loading on knee is even higher than for a normal gait (approximately 16.7%) and somewhat different (having two distinct maxima instead of a smooth variation; also the active cycle is narrow than for normal gait) characteristic for a stepped gait as reported for cerebral palsy patients [47]. Also, one could see that kinematics data show some increased activity when compared with the normal gait patterns.

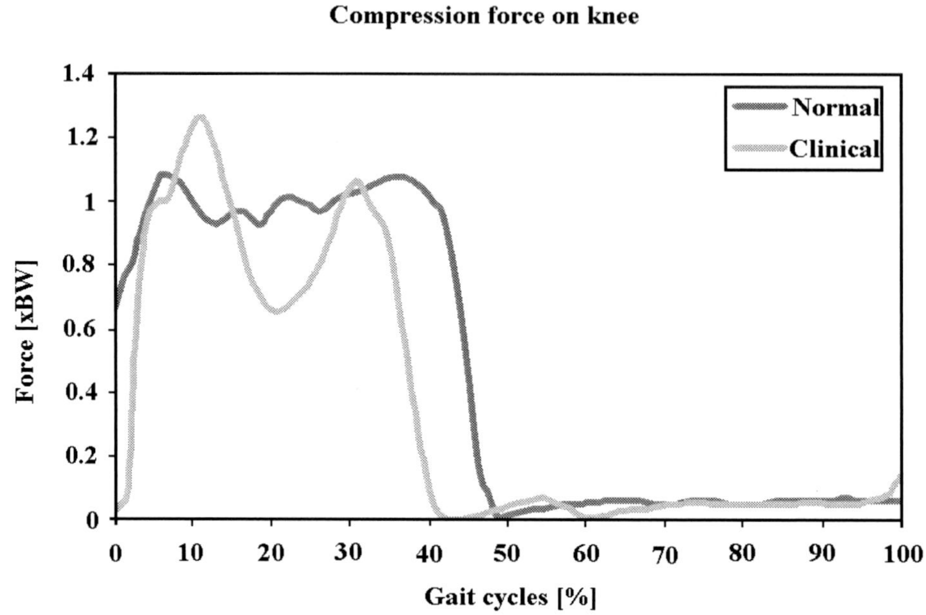

Figure 24. Compression force on the knee joint.

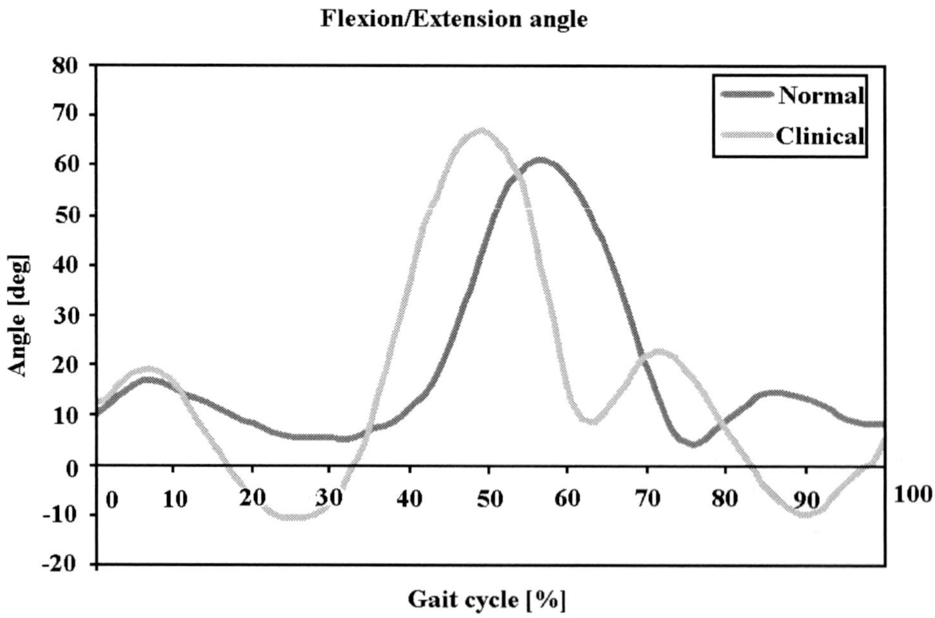

Figure 25. Compression of flexion/ extension angle.

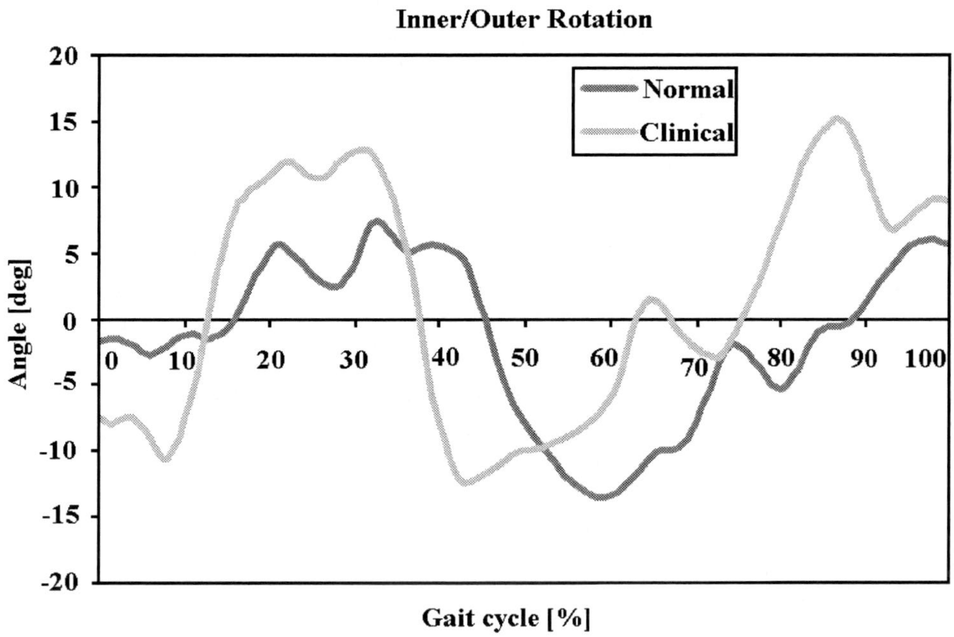

Figure 26. Compression of the dynamics of knee joint.

Conclusion

A method utilising finite element analysis (FEA) for evaluating the contact mechanism in an artificial knee joint with a summation technique based on a damage estimator was successfully used to predict the areas where the damage is likely to occur. Based on the study described above, one can formulate several conclusions.

First, the fatigue wear was identified as the main phenomenon responsible for the polyethylene tibial insert failure. Clinical studies show that even tibial parts that are retrieved for other reasons (implant loosening, misalignment, etc.) presented markers of fatigue wear (cracks in the subsurface, wear pits, delamination, and loss of large pieces of polyethylene).

The cumulative nature of the fatigue wear phenomenon requires a qualitative and quantitative evaluation of the transfer of loadings through the joint and a summation technique that is relevant for the variety of the human activities. The first part was assessed by a combination of dynamic finite element analyses of the joint contact mechanism. For the second part, we assumed that normal walking, stair ascending and stair descending were the regular activities with a dominant impact on the phenomenon. For the all three activities, the finite element analyses were performed, and a damage score was computed. Finally, a cumulative damage score (that accounts for all three activities) was determined and the areas where the fatigue wear is likely to occur were identified.

From the distribution of the cumulative damage score, one can see that the areas that may be damaged are located medially in the median and posterior regions of the tibial insert. Although the activities of stair ascending and descending generate a higher contact pressure due to the increased frequency, normal walking is still dominant.

A closer look at the distribution of the damage score reveals that the maximum damage is not likely to occur at the contact surface, but, rather, in the subsurface. The presence of maximum values in an area where other studies [31] have identified an increase of the percentage crystallinity and the presence of a subsurface oxidation peak induced by γ irradiation and the ageing of the prosthesis could be an explanation for the early delamination of the polyethylene inserts. We intend to extend this study in two directions: first – the contact mechanism would be improved by considering the polyethylene viscoelastoplasticity and a better friction mechanism (accounting for the dependency of the friction coefficient on the contact pressure and the velocity of the relative movement between the joint surfaces); second – the summation technique should be extended to a large area of activities, allowing for a better estimation of the influence of the frequency of the loadings.

In the case of total knee prostheses, previous studies reveal that there is a strong correlation between the wearing rate and the contact pressure. Therefore, the wearing phenomenon will be not a constant rate phenomenon for the same activity or across activities. The distribution of the contact pressure was dynamically evaluated by non-linear FEA that simulated the active cycle of normal walking, stairs ascending and stairs descending. The maxima of the contact pressure are plotted for each activity. A summation technique was adopted to evaluate the wear rate across activities.

The adopted method used a newly defined parameter, namely, the wear geometrical descriptor, which is a good estimator of the distribution of worn areas across the contact interface. By integrating this descriptor over the entire joint contact surface, the wear volumetric rate was obtained. The resulting value (28.17 $mm^3/10^6$ cycles) is in concordance with the values determined from experimental tests performed with special knee joint simulators. Appreciating the wear of the tibial tray of total knee prosthesis is very difficult. Measuring the wear becomes more challenging due to polyethylene's considerable yield. It is also difficult to establish the value of the wear factor, because the measuring volume of material removed is also complicated to do. At the moment, appreciating the wear of the tibial tray through simulation is generally done using qualitative methods, based on the microscopic investigation of the wear imprints. The initial polishing of the polyethylene's contact surface is a sign certifying the adhesive nature of wear. The tests carried out for a different number of cycles prove that the wear rate of the γ irradiated and air convection aged disks was greater in the beginning, decreasing afterwards and getting stabilized around the values of the wear rates for not irradiated specimens. The wear rate of the γ irradiated and aged 10 mm thick disks is about twice as for those that were not irradiated. The wear rate for 5 mm aged disks is greater than that of similar disks, with a 10 mm thickness. The results obtained lead to the conclusion that many clinically reported failures of the tibial tray are caused by the mechanisms of adhesive and fatigue wear.

The results obtained here shows that for an accurate estimation of damaging of tibial inserts under cyclic loading must account for the differences between generally used loading functions (from literature) and the real loadings. For clinical cases when abnormal walking occurs, the method described here estimates better because incorporates the specific loadings for each patient.

References

[1] Frey, M., Riener, R., Michas, C., Regenfelder, F., Burgkart, R. Elastic properties of an intact and ACL-ruptured knee joint: Measurement, mathematical modelling, and haptic rendering, *J. of Biomechanics*, 39, 1371–1382, 2006.

[2] Zheng, N., Fleisig, G.S., Escamilla, R.F., Barrentine, S.W., 1998. An analytical model of the knee for estimation of internal forces during exercise, *J. of Biomechanics*, 31, 963–967, 1998.

[3] Wilson, D.R., Feikes, J.D., O'Conner, J.J., 1998. Ligaments and articular contact guide passive knee flexion. *J. of Biomechanics*, 31, 1127–1136, 1998.

[4] Feikes, J.D., O'Conner, J.J., Zavatsky, A.B., 2000. A constraint-based approach to modelling the mobility of the human knee joint, *J. of Biomechanics,* 36, 125–129, 2000.

[5] Wismans, J., Veldpaus, F., Janssen, J., Huson, A., Struben, P., A three-dimensional mathematical model of the knee-joint, *J. of Biomechanics*, 13, 677–685, 1980.

[6] Engin, A.E., Moeinzadeh, M.H., *Modeling of human joint structure*, AFAMRL Report, AFAMRL-TR-81-117, 1982.

[7] Blankvoort, L., Kuiper, J.H., Huiskes, R., Grootenboer, H.J., Articular contact in a three-dimensional model of the knee. *J. of Biomechanics* 24, 1019–1031, 1991.

[8] Tumer, S.T., Engin, A.E., Three-Body segment dynamic model of the human knee. *J. of Biomechanical Engineering ASME Transactions,* 115, 350–356, 1993.

[9] Delp, S.L., Loan, J.P., A graphic-based software system to develop and analyze models of musculoskeletal structures. *Computers in Biology and Medicine*, 25, 21–34, 1995.

[10] Ateshian, G.A., Soslowsky, L.J., Mow, V.C., Quantitation of articular surface topography and cartilage thickness in knee joints using strereophotogrammetry, *J. of Biomechanics,* 24, 761–776, 1991.

[11] Hirokawa, S., Three-dimensional mathematical model analysis of the patellofemoral joint, *J. of Biomechanics,* 24, 659–671, 1991.

[12] Scherrer, P.K., Hillberry, B.M., Piecewise mathematical representation of articular surfaces, *J. of Biomechanics*, 12, 301-311, 1979.

[13] Scherrer, P.K., *Determining the distance between the surface of two rigid bodies using parametric surface patches and an instrumental spatial linkage*, thesis, Purdue Univ., 1977.

[14] Hart, W.B., Computer graphics aid fuselage design. The leastsquares, *Engineering Materials and Design Institute*, 205–209, 1974.

[15] Almond, D.B., Numerical control for machining complex surfaces, *IBM Systems Journal*, 150–168, 1991.

[16] Hefzy, M.S., Yang, H., A three-dimensional anatomical model of the human patella-femoral joint, for the determination of the patello-femoral motion and contact characteristics, *J. of Biomechanical Engineering*, 15, 289–302, 1993.

[17] Ateshian, G.A., A B-spline least-squares surface-fitting method for articular surfaces of diarthrodial joints, *J. of Biomechanical Engineering* 115, 366-373, 1993.

[18] Bergmann, G., Deuretzbracher, G., Heller, M., Graichen, M., Rohlmann, A., Strauss, J., Duda, G.N. Hip contact forces and gait patterns from routine activities. *J. of Biomech*anics 34, pp. 859-71, 2001.

[19] Morlock, M., et al. Duration and frequencies of everyday activities in total hip patients, *J. of Biomechanics*., 34, pp. 873-881, 2001.

[20] Capitanu, L., Iarovici, A., Onisoru, J. Tribological behaviour of a Total Hip Prosthesis during normal walking active cycle, Proceedings of BALKANTRIB'05, Kragujevac, Serbia & Montenegro, pp. 317-323, 2005.

[21] Wang, A., Essner, A., Klein, R. Effect of contact stress on friction and wear of ultrahigh molecular weight polyethylene in total hip replacement, Proc. Inst. Mech. Eng. (part H), 215, pp. 133-139, 2001.

[22] Onisoru, J., Iarovici, A., Capitanu, L., Popescu, M.V. The contact mechanism between the artificial femoral head and UHMWPE cup, in Total Hip Prostheses, Proceedings of SISOM'05, Academic Press, Bucharest, 2005.

[23] Blunn G.W., Joshi A.B., Minns R.J. et all. Wear in retrieved condylar knee arthroplasties, *Journal of Arthroplasty*, 12, pp. 281-290, 1997.

[24] Wasielewski, R.C., Galante, J.O., Leighty, R.M., Natarajan, R.N., Rosenberg, A.G. Wear patterns on retrieved polyethylene tibial inserts and their relationship to technical considerations during total knee arthroplastes, *Clinical Orthopaedics*, 299, pp. 31–43, 1994.

[25] Knight, J.L., Gorai, P.A., Atwater, R.D., Grothaus, L. Tibial Polyethylene Failure After Primary Porous-coated Anatomic Total Knee Arthroplasty, *Journal of Arthroplasty*, 10, pp. 748-757, 1995.

[26] Heck, D.A., Clingman, J.K., Kettelkamp, D.G. Gross polyethylene failure in total knee arthroplasty. *Orthopedics*, 15, pp. 23-31, 1992.

[27] Engh, G.A., Dwyer, K.A., Hanes, C.K. Polyethlyene wear of metal-backed tibial components in total and unicompartmental knee prostheses, *J Bone Joint Surg*, 74B, pp. 9-17, 1992.

[28] Jones, S.M.G., Pinder, I.M., Moran, C.G., Malcolm, A.J. Polyethylene wear in uncemented knee replacements, *J Bone Joint Surg*, 74B, pp. 18-22, 1992.

[29] Kilgus, D.J., Moreland, J.R., Finerman, G.A., et al. Catastrophic wear of tibial polyethylene inserts, *Clin Orthop*, 273, pp. 223-231, 1991.

[30] Mintz, L., Tsao, A.K., McCrae, C.R., et al. The arthroscopic evaluation and characteristics of severe polyethylene wear in total knee arthroplasty. *Clin Orthop*, 273, pp. 215-222, 1991.

[31] Ries, M.D., Bellare, A., Livingston, B.J., Cohen, R.E., Spector, M. Early Delamination of a Hylamer-M tibial insert. *Journal of Arthroplasty*, 10, pp. 974- 976, 1995.

[32] Oonishi, H., Kim, S.C., Kyomoto, M., Iwamoto, M., Ueno, M. PE wear in ceramic/PE bearing surface in total knee arthroplasty; Clinical experiences of more than 24 years, 2006, Bioceramics and Alternative Bearings in Joint Arthroplasty, 11-th BIOLOX Symposium

[33] Onisoru, J., Capitanu, L., Iarovici, A., 2006, Failure of a tibial insert of a total knee prosthesis due to fatigue wear, *Buletinul Institutului Politehnic din Iasi,* Tomul LII (LVI), Fasc. 6A, ACME 2006/1, pp.333-340

[34] Lewis, G. Properties of cross-linked ultra-high-molecular-weight polyethylene, *Biomaterials*, 22, pp. 371-401, 2001.

[35] Taylor, S.J.G., Walker, P.S. Forces and moments telemetered from two distal femoral replacements during various activities, *Journal of Biomechanics*, 34, pp. 839-848, 2001

[36] Villa, T., Migliavacca, F., Gastaldi, D., Colombo, M., Pietrabissa, R. Contact stresses and fatigue life in a knee prosthesis: comparison between in vitro measurements and computational simulation. *Journal of Biomechanics* 37, pp. 45-53, 2004.

[37] Sathasivam, S., Walker, P.S. The conflicting requirements of laxity and conformity in total knee replacement, *Journal of Biomechanics*, 32, pp. 239-247, 1999.

[38] Onisoru, J., Capitanu, L., Iarovici, A., Popescu, M. A method for predicting the wear of the artificial joints, *Journal of Biomechanics*, Volume 39 (Suppl 1), S141, 2006.

[39] Saikko, V., Ahlroos, T., Calonius, O. A three –axis wear simulator with ball-on-flat contact. *Wear* 249, pp. 310-315, 2001

[40] Archard, J.F. Contact and Rubbing of flat Surfaces, *J.Appl. Phys.*, 24, 1953, pp.438-455.

[41] Yoshikawa, T., Zheng, X.Z. Coordinated Dynamic Hybrid Position/Force Control for Multiple Robot Manipulators Handling On Constrained Object, *Intern. Journal of Robotics Research*, 12, No. 3, June 1993, pp. 219-230

[42] Mason M. Compliance and force control for computer controlled manipulators, The MIT Press, Cambridge, MA, 1982, ch.5, pp.373-404

[43] Denavit, J. Hartenberg, R.B., *A kinematic notation for lower-pair mehcanism based on matrices*, *ASME J. Appl. Mechanics*, 23, 1955, pp.215-221

[44] Joly, L.D., Andriot, C., Hayward, V. *Mechanical Analogic in Hybrid Position/Force Control"*, IEEE Albuquerque, New Mexico, 1997, pp. 835-840

[45] Vladareanu, L., Peterson, T. New Concepts for the Real Time Control of Robots by Open Architecture Systems, *Machine Building*, vol.55, ISSN 0573-7419 no.11, 2003

[46] Vladareanu, L. *The Open Achitecture (OAH) Control in Real Time for the Contour Robots* – AMSE 2003- International Conference of Management and Technology MT'2003, Habana, Cuba, 2003, pp. 131-139

[47] Vaughan, C.L., Davis, B.L., O'Connor, J.C., *Dynamics of Human Gait,* 2nd Edition, 1999, Kiboho Publishers, South Africa

In: New Developments in Knee Prosthesis Research
Editor: Janice Stewart
ISBN: 978-1-63482-700-3

Chapter 4

The Use of Finite Element Modeling to Improve Biomechanical Research on Knee Prosthesis

Silvia Pianigiani[1*] ***and Bernardo Innocenti***[2]
[1]IRCCS Istituto Ortopedico Galeazzi, Milano, Italy
[2]BEAMS Department Université Libre de Bruxelles, Bruxelles, Belgium

Abstract

Biomechanical numerical models in orthopedic research are currently becoming more and more frequent, complex and comprehensive. In this context, finite element analysis of biomechanical models has consistently increased in the last decades. The growing trend in the use of such numerical technique is indeed strongly correlated with the increasing and the easiest access to computational resources and, parallel to this, with the development of more sophisticated data handling algorithms. In fact, looking to the past, the use of finite element analysis in the field of biomechanics was mainly limited to simplistic approaches, such as bi-dimensional models, considering mainly linear analyses, and investigation of single structures or tissue types only. Nowadays, fully three-dimensional, nonlinear, multi-structures and tissues, and even multi-joint systems, can be also easily implemented in the simulation. More specifically, for a knee with an implant (e.g., total knee arthroplasty (TKA), unicondilar knee arthroplasty (UKA) or patello-femoral joint), the model aims to replicate the behavior of three-dimensional biological structures, like bones, cartilage and ligaments, coupled with non-biological knee components made of different synthetic materials.

An additional complexity in knee modeling is provided by the huge variability inherent to the field. This variability is due to the vast range of different kinematics and contact forces that could be induced by the variety of prosthesis designs, in different patients, and under specific motor tasks.

Due to the multiplicity of these aspects, the use of finite element modeling is of foremost importance; in fact, it allows to obtain qualitative guesses and qualitative data

* Corresponding author: Silvia Pianigiani, silvia.pianigiani84@gmail.com.

that cannot be provided by any other method (such as in-vitro experimental tests or gait analysis) such as the stresses distribution for bone and prosthesis components under different conditions, and contact forces interactions, both for generic and patient-specific solutions. These outputs, coupled with clinical outputs, allow to relate, for example, stress changes, from the physiological to a knee with a prosthesis and to a bone mineral density changes in the patients, allowing to formulate possible answers to common unsolved clinical questions.

An added value derived by the use of finite element analysis is the possibility to characterize performances of prosthesis designs in restoring knee functions and maintaining long-term mechanical integrity for different patients and in agreement with different surgeon requests.

In more general terms, the use of finite element modeling in the understanding of knee prosthesis biomechanics is fundamental to answer clinical questions, to improve and predict clinical outputs, to provide more surgeon-friendly guidelines and, last but not least, to improve TKA success and avoid critical situations.

This modeling procedure can help bridging the gap between surgeons and engineers, aiming in the improving of the biomechanical research on knee prosthesis.

Introduction

When there is a degenerative knee condition, a knee prosthesis is a possible, and usually most common, solution to restore the patient's condition [1].

From the very first knee prosthesis design up to now, multiple solutions were designed. All these designs were defined on different theories mainly based on the actual knee biomechanical knowledge at that time, in terms of anatomy and functionality.

Even if there are several proposed solutions, in the last decade, a need for different features in knee prostheses design is still manifested. In fact, several patients still complain bad experiences after a knee arthroplasty, or they are generally not happy [2,3]. Surgeons and industries are therefore searching for different solutions, both in terms of designs and surgical techniques, to restore and improve the patient's knee functionality.

Among the several causes of patients' discontent, changes in the potential patient's profile through the years must be considered [4]. Actually, the patient's average age is decreasing and so the expected activities to be performed change as well [5-8]. Moreover, nowadays, also older patients have high expectations after a knee arthroplasty [9,10].

The high expectations for TKA performances are, however, discordant with the highly invasive procedure for the native knee that happens when a knee arthroplasty is implanted. First, it needs a quite large scar to be performed. Then, several tissues are cut and some of them could suffer consequent stitches. When the knee prosthesis is finally positioned, a significant change in the knee may affect both geometries, which could be similar, but not equal to the patient's native ones, and, even more changes are induced by the different synthetic materials, that are harder and more rigid than the native ones, for i.e., considering the soft cartilage and meniscus that are usually replaced with polyethylene-based structures. Friction coefficients may be consequently different, and all these considered aspects could reasonably induce a change in the joint performance.

To completely or even partially address these aspects, different solutions could be envisioned to improve knee prostheses, both in terms of improved designs and the synthesis of new-generated materials and of research in innovative surgical techniques. Nevertheless, whatever is the chosen aspect to be improved, superior information about knee behaviour must be nowadays still provided.

To be able to better analyse and predict the 3D behaviour of a knee, native or post knee arthroplasty, the use of numerical modelling is so fundamental as unique tool or to be complementary to experimental and clinical research.

Different methodologies are nowadays carried out to perform research on knee behaviour. When clinical research cannot answer to pressing questions, experimental procedures, also performed on human knee specimens, are considered optimal to closely investigate how a knee behaves under several conditions including the presence of knee implants [11-13]. Clinical research is mainly based on during-surgery observations or non-invasive analysis on patients' records during the follow-up. Unfortunately, clinical observations often start after a group of patients presents some post-surgery related issues or in case a particular pathology is already present. Furthermore, several limitations could also affect the experimental procedures, such as the limited number of simulated boundary conditions, and, generally, the low amount of analysed specimens for specific configurations, which are sometimes retrospective and/or not randomized. Moreover, in-vivo analyses, such as gait analyses and fluoroscopy, are also useful to better subdivide particular knee behaviour in categories in order to detect particular pathologies; yet they are still affected by limitations in the extracted outputs, in the limited sample size of the study, and the accuracy that can be achieved.

On the other hand, the use of numerical modelling can solve several of the limitations of the experimental procedures, although, before concluding outputs could be considered for clinical practice, models must be before validated. Validation is usually performed by comparing numerical outputs with experimental data when the same configuration under the same boundary conditions is replicated.

As a general definition, models are conceptual constructions which allow formulation and testing of hypotheses. The model parameters can be easily altered both in the black box and for the building box models.

In the last decades, the use of computational modelling exponentially increased [14] thanks also to the improving and the easiest access of computational resources and, in parallel, the raise of more sophisticated data handling algorithms.

In fact, looking into the past, the use of finite element analysis in biomechanics was mainly limited to a simplistic approach, such as bi-dimensional models [15], considering mainly linear analyses, and investigating only single structures or tissue types [16]. Nowadays, fully three-dimensional, nonlinear, multi-structures and tissues, and even multi-joint systems can be also simulated. The latter models allow applying different load conditions and specific patients' geometries.

The use of finite element analysis is therefore allowing to comprehensively analyse different outputs for several conditions, also for deformable structures, such as in patient-specific native joints [17]. Another added value in using finite element analysis for knee understanding is the possibility to characterize the performances of different knee prosthesis designs in restoring knee function and maintaining long-term mechanical integrity for specific patients' and surgeons' requests.

More generally, the use of this numerical approach is nowadays essential to generate question-specific models and to provide the missing knowledge in order to answer clinical questions, to improve and predict clinical outputs, helping industry in generating new knee devices and surgeon-friendly instrumentation and, generally, to improve research about knee behaviour knowledge.

In this chapter, an overview on how generating a knee model with a prosthetic device will be provided in order to understand its feasibility, the possible features, advantages, errors and limitations with respect to other research methods. Moreover, some reported models and their applications will be also briefly presented and discussed.

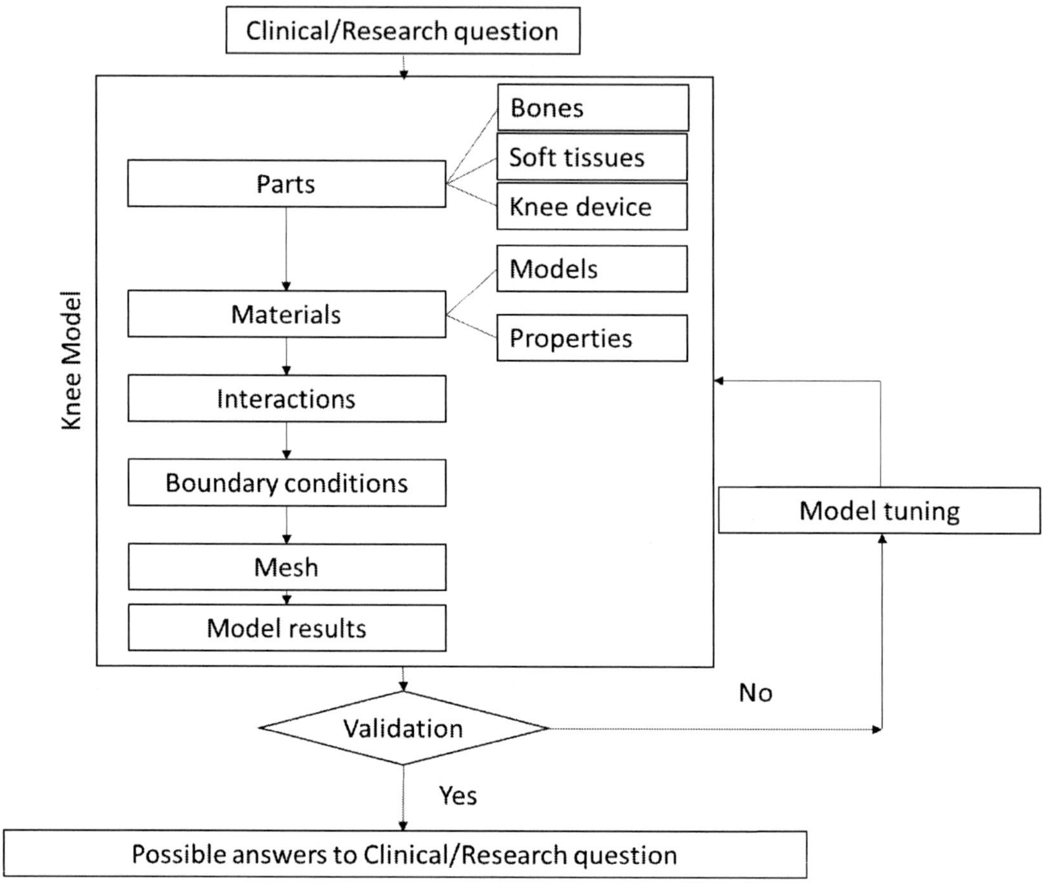

Figure 1. How obtaining a validated model of a specific knee system to help in replying to a clinical or research question. The model is generated, based on specific requests, as an isolated system from the rest of the world by using specific boundaries. The system is conceptually reduced under simplifying assumptions. Consequently, the model results will present limitations valid only in the regimes where the assumptions are valid. So, the model should be validated by using experimental data for the same used boundary conditions. In absence of an acceptable match between numerical and experimental outputs, the model should be corrected for one or all its steps. When the model is validated, its outputs can be used as possible explanations to the formulated clinical/research question.

The flow chart styled in Figure 1 will be followed to describe how obtaining a validated model of a specific knee system to help in replying to a clinical or research question.

Model Geometries Definition

In order to completely define the parts that generate the model assembly, several preliminary considerations should be discussed.

First, the model could be general or patient-specific. If the model should be used for general knee behaviour outputs, the model should implement standard bone shapes, dimensions and relative positions; moreover, this information should be used to generate reference coordinate systems based on the standards [18] for the consequent knee behaviour interpretation. On the other hand, when the analysis of a patient-specific knee is needed, the model should implement patient's bone geometries, and relative orientations should be known to re-create the patient's configuration. Usually, in case complete patient's information is available, CT scans are used to reconstruct the femur, tibia, fibula and patella geometries and to find the reference landmarks [11] in order to characterize the useful knee axes and relative positions of bones. Moreover, if needed, CT scans can be used in order to localize the main soft tissues bone attachments. If patient's images are not available, morphing techniques can be eventually used to obtain close to patient's bone shapes. On the other hand, nowadays, MRI scans can be also used to obtain accurate long bones reconstructions. MRIs are a good alternative to obtain patient-specific data not involving ionizing radiation. Furthermore, when soft tissues, such as cartilage and menisci, should be also implemented, MRI scans become almost fundamental in order to evaluate their geometries and conditions. MRIs are then also a useful key in order to reconstruct the ligaments geometries or to understand possible pathologies, such as ligaments ruptures, to be replicated. Several software allow nowadays to manually or more automatically reconstruct all these structures.

To be more comprehensive and realistic, the knee model should not be limited to the bone structures, but should include also the knee envelop. Its contribution is not easy to be replicated due to the big amount of soft tissues structures involved, consequently in the most common practice only the main ligaments are replicated as single or multi bundles elements that can be mono, bi or tri-dimensionally reproduced in the finite element analyses, [19]. The main ligaments are positioned in the model basing on the previously defined landmarks. Regarding the muscles, they are usually not included in the knee model as indipendent parts, rather their action is simulated as applied forces (see boundary conditions section).

Then, once the bone geometries are selected or defined, and the ligaments modelling approach is chosen, another important consideration must be formulated regarding the kind of analysis that should be performed.

In fact, the obtained model can be used for an understanding of physiological conditions or can be adopted to investigate pathologic conditions or different knee prosthesis solutions. If the research question is about native knees (both physiological and pathological conditions), all the above mentioned structures (i.e., bones and all the soft-tissues) should be considered in the model. On the other hand, in performing an analysis that includes a knee prosthesis, the components of the analysed prosthesis should be also included in the model, and the relative position to the knee bones and structures should be replicated following the manufacturer's guidelines, or specific configurations in interest. That could mean that, dependently on the analysed knee design, several native knee structures should not be considered in the final model. For example, in the case of a total knee arthroplasty, menisci, cartilages, and eventually the cruciate ligaments are not needed in the model.

Furthermore, even several geometry optimizations can be performed dependently on the requested outputs, in order to let the final model have only the geometrical features useful for the dedicated analysis, and so optimizing the computational cost of the final simulation. For example, if the simulation is meant to understand the interactions between prosthesis components under specific conditions, bone geometries can be removed from the final model after recording their useful landmarks and contributions. Moreover, in this case, the femoral component is usually considered as a rigid skin instead of a solid body in order to reduce even more the final computing time during the model simulation.

Once all needed geometries have been defined and eventually optimized in their shape features to satisfy the research question criteria, the final parts assembly can be so generated. From the reference generated assembly, some model parameters can be altered in order to generate several configurations and so to perform sensitivity analyses.

Material Models and Properties Implementation

Once the model assembly under specific modelling assumptions is defined, each part must be characterized by a material model with proper properties. To do so, literature-proved data or in-vivo measurements by imaging analysis can be used. In fact, direct in-vivo measurements on the patient are not usually possible to reliably characterize bones' and soft tissues materials, but patients' information, such as gender, age, and images data, can be an added valid support to identify the best matching material models and properties characterizing the patient, based on literature.

In a macroscopic model of the knee, the bone can be considered as a homogeneous material, or mainly subdivided in its cortical and trabecular structures using transverse isotropic model and isotropic model, respectively [20]. The properties of the bones structure can be varied in a range to simulate from healthy to pathologic conditions, such as osteoporosis, for which material properties can degrade (up to 66% for trabecular bone [21]).

Regarding the soft tissues, multiple approaches are reported in literature for menisci, cartilage and ligaments. Unfortunately, due to several aspects, data confusion is quite often present when performing a literature search about material behaviour of all these soft tissues [19]. Different concerns about their real behaviour have been reported in several papers in the years. This brings the choice of the soft tissue material models and properties to be, possibly, the most difficulty definable and weakest point of a knee model. Usually, to simplify the model, also depending on the computational time requests, and due to the lack of information, all these materials are chosen to be modelled as linear elastic or quasi-linear elastic materials and following literature data most cited paper for defining their individual properties [19]. That brings many models to be patient-specific more for the geometrical reconstructions than for the material modelling part.

Despite the fact that defining the proper materials for the patients' structure is complex, and that the results could partially account for the realistic tissues behaviour, replicating the synthetic materials with which the prostheses components are made of is less intricate. Generally, the manufacturer provides the main features of used materials for a specific knee prosthesis design. This brings the developers of the knee model a key in searching the best material model and properties. Usually, metallic knee components are replicated as linear elastic or rigid components, while the plastic components can be assumed to be linear elastic, or, more specifically, their plastic behaviour could be replicated. If cement needs to be considered, it can be replicated as linear elastic plastic material, and material properties can be obtained from the manufacturer or literature; so bone-cement interactions could be also implemented [22].

Once materials are modelled, the proper friction coefficient should be also considered between each material couple. This friction coefficient should also simulate the presence of the synovial joint liquid.

Thus, after a meticulous material characterization research for the specific knee model to be developed, all the materials and relative friction coefficients can be associated with relative components, and the final assembly is now ready to be implemented with interactions and boundary conditions to replicate a specific task.

Applied Boundary Conditions

When developing a knee model to be used for finite element analysis, specific interactions should be considered among the structures to simulate the real boundary conditions. For example, correct interactions need to be set among components that are, or are going to be, in contact during the simulated motion.

For the ligaments, the pre-strain and, especially when they are modelled as tri-dimensional structures, special interactions should be applied to replicate/simulate the wrapping of these soft tissues around the bone structures. Moreover, for the cartilages and the meniscus, different degrees of freedom can be replicated with selected interactions on the entire or partial geometries.

A commonly used solution is to rigidly link some structures to reference points in which some of the boundary conditions can be applied. This is the case when simulating the action of the muscles that are usually rigidly connected to the bone structures, or directly to the TKA components, and their action is simulated with applied forces on the involved model parts.

The remaining boundary conditions to be set are related to all the forces and movements inputs in order to replicate a real motor task, including also the embedding of some of the degrees of freedom. The performed task can be statically or dynamically replicated, and generally can be force or displacement controlled. Each of these assumptions has proper advantages/disadvantages. For i.e., in dynamic simulations a displacement controlled movement, for example with data collected from in-vivo analysis, could better converge if inputs are accurate and they do not generate too many deformed geometries. However, usually dynamic simulations last longer than static ones and are not necessary if only a specific task segment should be analysed.

Forces and kinematics inputs can have different origins in literature. They can depend on different reference systems or can be obtained with different procedures. They should nevertheless be all coherent for the specific simulated task when selected as boundary conditions for the model. These inputs could be patient-specific, from previous gait-analysis registrations or instrumented prostheses data, or could be more general. To be more standardized, standards reported in the literature are usually used, such as the standard curves that are implemented to test life expectancy of the prostheses components.

Finite Element Features

Once the previous steps are defined, the finite element model is not yet ready to simulate certain requested configurations. A fundamental point of finite element analysis is to give a mesh to the structures to be analysed. That means to subdivide the object in little elements. The properties and the governing relationships are assumed over these elements, and are expressed mathematically at specific points called nodes.

Regarding the knee joint, its native bone and soft tissues shapes are complex and continuous, but also devices designs present particular shapes in order to be adapted to the anatomical environment. Giving a mesh to such geometries means going from a continuous to a discrete spatial approximation of the parts of interest. For this reason a good mesh is necessary, but not sufficient, to have the results of the simulation in good agreement with the real knee behaviour. However, an approximation of the reality is anyway performed.

In order to obtain the best mesh, i.e., leading to the least possible approximations, several options are possible in meshing a component. These options, such as different element types that allow different degree of distortion, and sizes, can be selected depending on several aspects, such as the dimension and the regularity in the shape of a specific part, the expected accuracy of the outputs and the available computational time.

Usually, mesh convergence tests are performed to verify if a selected element type and the chosen size are the optimal to mesh an object. The accuracy of the outputs, achieved by this couple of selected options to mesh the part in interest, is compared with the data outputs obtained by changing, e.g., the size of the chosen element type to give the mesh. If the accuracy of the outputs is independent of the mesh size, the biggest mesh size is so selected. The convergence test allows in this way to select the minimum number of elements necessary for a specific part in order to obtain a prefixed accuracy in the outputs. This is useful to justify future requested computational time and avoid unnecessary increment in simulation time and resource consumption.

Output Requests and Analysis

Finite element analysis of a knee model allows the determination of several outputs. As example, bone and prosthesis kinematics, implant contact forces and contact pressures, bone stresses and ligament strains are some of the most requested outputs determined in finite element model to understand knee behaviour under specific configurations.

Not all the outputs should be requested for all the simulations. Usually different requests are formulated dependently on the clinical/research questions under the obtained knee model.

According to the parts of the knee assembly in analysis, stresses outputs, can be requested to understand femoral component-polyethylene insert interfaces, tibia bone stress maps dependent on the cement layer. Contact forces and pressure could be an interesting output to be analysed, or the post-cam mechanism in a specific posterior stabilized knee design. On the other hand, kinematic outputs are fundamental to understand wheter a specific design movement could be compared to physiological behaviour under the same task boundary conditions. Strain outputs are useful to understand soft tissues behaviour, especially for ligaments, for instance when, for the same patient, different knee implants are considered, or in possible mal-aligned configurations.

When all these aspects are considered, a user has his own model obtained under specific considerations for the parts included, the materials of each component, the interactions, the boundary conditions, the accuracy and the expected simulation time, and, finally, the outputs he needs to answer a specific clinical/research question.

A first check should be to evaluate wheter the obtained outputs have a real meaning. In fact, the expected range of movement for different directions are known from literature, at least for the physiological conditions and some of the prosthesis designs; and this basilar knowledge, together with the magnitude of the obtained contact forces and pressures, should be evaluated before even proceeding with the model validation. If the model exits with not comprehensible behaviour, simple tests, such as a compressive test, should be verified with theoretical models in order to evaluate the model bugs and, eventually correct them properly.

Model Validation

Regardless the type of developed knee model, a proper model validation must be performed before the obtained data can be safely and trustfully used by clinicians and industry, in order to help them with the surgical practice or in improving knee designs features.

The validation of a knee model can be based on experimental studies performed on knee specimens that replicate the same specimen geometries, boundary conditions and, eventually, knee prosthesis design. Also in-vivo tests performed with instrumented prostheses or gait-lab analysis can be used to compare the model outputs for similar boundary conditions. Other studies published in literature can be integrated to further compare the obtained knee trends; however particular care should be given in understanding wheter the studies are at all comparable before analysing the outputs.

Whatever the bases of comparison, the achieved outputs under the numerical method should be analysed and compared to one of the previously mentioned information. In case of outputs divergences, a careful ponderation of possible correlations of these outputs differences to procedural errors, hypotheses and limitations should be performed formulating acceptable expected errors. If the model does not respect the validation criteria, a tuning of the model is recommended in order to improve it and make it reliable. This step is important not only to calibrate the model with real outputs, but also to verify how and how much the model is sensible to variations of its input parameters.

Once all these aspects are verified, the developed knee model can be considered validated and so also trustable for clinical and industrial advices. Moreover, once the model is so validated, it can be used also to simulate other configurations under similar boundary conditions carrying on sensitivity analyses. For instance, the same motor task can be simulated, by changing the material properties of the bones to simulate the effects in the outputs due to pathologies such as osteoporosis.

Example Cases

Following the previous indications, different knee models can be obtained. More and more accurate finite element knee models can be found in the literature.

Among the validated ones, knee models have been developed for different aims.

For example, Innocenti et al. [23] generated a validated knee model to understand the UKA behavior under compression boundary conditions. This study was validated with experimental tests that replicate the same geometry and boundary conditions of the numerical model. This study clearly demonstrate the importance of the integration of collateral ligaments in the model for its stability and correspondance to real behavior. In fact, only through this feature there was excellent agreement among numerical and experimental results.

Another paper [21] presents a solution to unsolved clinical questions regarding the risk of fracture in femoral bone where total hip and revision knee prosthesis are simultaneously present. The numerical model was able to implement and investigate the effect of several lengths for the stem of the revision TKA coupled with a hip prosthesis. The model has been loaded for different configurations simulating walking and falling motor tasks. By analyzing the bone stresses outputs, the study demonstrates that there is a relation between the relative distance of the hip and knee stems and the potential risk of fracture. This relation was also demonstrated for healthy and osteoporotic bone quality. Consequently, this work uses finite element simulation to provide clinical guidelines.

Then, Catani et al. [24] coupled in-vivo fluoroscopic data with FEA in order to improve a clinical methodology and allowing the investigation understanding from such in-vivo obtained information, therefore improving clinical measurements. In fact, during fluoroscopy it is not possible to directly measure metal-polyethylene contact. Yet by coupling this information with FEA, this work was the first to analyze the in-vivo tibio-femoral contact and also post-cam contact interaction during daily activities. The numerical outputs, in this case, have been validated with robotic simulations outputs.

Finally, in another work [25] an implementation of patello-femoral wear was described in order to be able to predict polyethylene wear under several configurations. As for the tibio-femoral interaction, polyethylene wear can be measured with experimental techniques using wear simulators. This procedure is time consuming and expensive. Conversely the wear model was calibrated and validated for the implementation of the patella-femoral wear and it can be used for several applications, such as investigating wear for different configurations.

General Discussion

The value of finite element numerical modelling for understanding knee behaviour is considerable. Like in other fields, literature proves how such methodology is becoming complementary to other research techniques in order to obtain improved knowledge about knee behaviour under different conditions.

The use of finite element analysis allows obtaining several answers that cannot be achieved with any other method (such as the stresses distribution for bone and prosthesis components under different conditions and also for patient-specific solutions). These outputs, coupled with clinical outputs, allow relating, for example, the stress changes, from the physiological to a knee with prosthesis, to a bone mineral density change in the patients, letting to formulate a possible reply to common clinical questions.

Native knee understanding is still a hot topic in orthopaedics, but also for knees with an implant the knee model aims to replicate the behaviour of three-dimensional biological structures, like bones, cartilage and ligaments, coupled with non-biological knee components made of different synthetic materials. An added value derived by the use of finite element analysis is to characterize performances of prosthesis designs in restoring knee functions and maintaining long-term mechanical integrity for different patients' and surgeons' requests.

Through the years, knee models have become more complex and comprehensive. The increasing trend in the use of such technique is indeed strongly correlated with the increase of and the easiest access to computational resources and, in the parallel, the development of more sophisticated data handling algorithms.

Defining a finite element model of the knee joint is not unique. Different complexity levels could be achieved according to different research questions and the outputs accuracy that should be reached. Levels of complexity in knee modelling are provided by the vast range of different kinematics and contact forces that could be achieved by different patients, by different prosthesis designs and under different motor tasks.

General limitations regarding knee models are especially correlated with assumptions in the model definition, at all the levels, from geometry definition, passing through material till boundary conditions and mesh. For these reasons, a comparison that allows a validation of a model must be provided in order to efficiently and trustfully apply the result to real practice.

Common sense believes that the best characteristic of knee modelling is to be faster and cheaper with respect to other research approaches, such as experimental tests on knee specimens. Actually, developing a validated finite element model of the knee could be time consuming. Yet it is true that, once the model is developped and validated, it can quickly produce several outputs for different configurations that, otherwise, could be not replicable with other methodologies, or could be more expensive and anyway limited, considering several possible variable inputs, than following the numerical approach.

As with any use of finite element analysis, the practitioner must be an expert with good understanding of technical issues and some basic knowledge of the field of study in order to be able to understand if the developed model, with its own hypotheses and limitations, is valid. In the case of knee modelling, continuous support from clinicians should be provided from the correct formulation of the research question to the interpretation of obtaining results, to help in translating technical outputs into clinical guidelines.

Conclusion

The use of finite element modelling is indeed giving significant benefits in improving the knowledge of knee biomechanics and knee behaviour understanding. Improved achieved knee backgrounds allow providing answers and solutions to clinical paradoxes and to help industries in developing knee prostheses ever closer to replicate physiologic knee movements and adapted for patient-specific configurations.

This modeling procedure can help bridging the gap between surgeons and engineers aiming in the improving of biomechanical research on knee prosthesis.

References

[1] S M Kurtz, K L Ong, E Lau, M Widmer, M Maravic, E Gómez-Barrena, F de Pina, V Manno, M Torre, W L Walter, R de Steiger, R G Geesink, M Peltola, Röder. "International survey of primary and revision total knee replacement". *Int Orthop.* 2011,35:1783-9.

[2] R B Bourne, B M Chesworth, A M Davis, N N Mahomed, K D J Charron. "Patient Satisfaction after Total Knee Arthroplasty: Who is Satisfied and Who is Not?". *Clin Orthop Relat Res.* 2010,46:57–63.

[3] R M Nunley,D Nam, K R Berend, AV Lombardi, D A Dennis, C J Della Valle, R L Barrack. "New total knee arthroplasty designs: do young patients notice?". *Clin Orthop Relat Res.* 2015,473:101-8.

[4] AV Lombardi, R M Nunley, K R Berend, E L Ruh, J C Clohisy,W G Hamilton, C J Della Valle, J Parvizi, R L Barrack. "Do patients return to work after total knee arthroplasty?". *Clin Orthop Relat Res.* 2014,472:138-46.

[5] R Bisschop, R W Brouwer, J Van Raay. "Total Knee Arthroplasty in Younger Patients: A 13-year Follow-up Study". *Orthopedics.* 2010,33:12.

[6] F S Hossain, S Patell, M A Fernandez, S Konan, F S Haddad. "A performance based patient outcome score for active patients following total knee arthroplasty". *Osteoarthritis Cartilage.* 2013,21:51-9.

[7] W J Long, C D Brycce, C S Hollenbeak, R W Benner, W N Scott. "Total Knee Replacement in Young, Active Patients: Long-Term Follow-up and Functional Outcome. A Concise Follow-up of a Previous Report". *J Bone Joint Surg Am.* 2014,96:e159.

[8] D R Diduch, J N Insall, W N Scott, G L Scuderi, D Font-RodriguezClohisy, W G Hamilton, C J Della Valle, J Parvizi, R L Barrack. "Total Knee Replacement in Young, Active Patients. Long-Term Follow-up and Functional Outcome". *J Bone Joint Surg Am.* 1997,79:575 -82.

[9] A F Mannion, S Kämpfen, U Munzinger,I Kramers-de Quervain. "The role of patient expectations in predicting outcome after total knee arthroplasty". *Arthritis Research&Therapy.* 2009,11:R139.

[10] P C Noble, M J Gordon, J M Weiss, R N Reddix, M A Conditt, K B Mathis. "Does total knee replacement restore normal knee function?". *Clin Orthop Relat Res.* 2005,431:157-65.

[11] J Victor, D Van Doninck, L Labey, B Innocenti, PM Parizel. "How precise can bony landmarks be determined on Ct scan of the knee?". *The Knee.* 2009,16:358-65.

[12] H D Delport. "Collateral Ligament Strain of the Human Knee Joint. Native and after Total Knee Arthroplasty". *Ph.D. thesis,* KU Leuven, Belgium, 2013.

[13] N Arnout, L Vanlommel, J Vanlommel, JP Luyckx, L Labey, B Innocenti, J Victor, J Bellemans. "Post-cam mechanics and tibiofemoral kinematics: a dynamic in vitro analysis of eight posterior-stabilized total knee designs". *Knee Surg Sports Traumatol Arthrosc.* 2014,doi:10.1007/s00167-014-3167-2.

[14] M Kazemi, Y Dabiri, L P Li. "Recent Advances in Computational Mechanics of the Human Knee Joint". Computational and Mathematical Methods in Medicine. 2013, Article ID 718423.

[15] R Huiskes, E Y S Chao. A survey of finite element analysis in orthopaedic biomechanics:the first decade. J Biomech. 1983,16:385-409.

[16] M S Hefzy, E S Grood. "Review of knee models". *Applied Mech Rev.* 1988,49:1-13.

[17] E Pena, B Calvo, M A Martinez, M Doblare. "A three-dimensional finite element analysis of the combined behaviour of ligaments and menisci in the healthy human knee joint". *J Biomech.* 2006,39:1686-1701.

[18] E S Grood, W J Suntay. "A joint coordinate system for the clinical description of three-dimensional motions: application to the knee". *J Biomech Eng.* 1983,105.

[19] F Galbusera, M Freutel, L Durselen, M D'Aiuto, D Croce, T Villa,V Sansone, B Innocenti. "Material models and properties in the finite elemnt analysis of knee ligaments: a literature review". *Frontiers in Bioeng and Biotech.* 2014,2:1-11.

[20] H P W van-Jonbergen, B Innocenti, G Luca Gervasi, L Labey, N Verdonschot. "Differences in the stress distribution in the distal femur between patellofemoral joint replacement and total knee replacement: a finite element study". *J Ortho Surg and Res.* 2012,7:1-9.

[21] M Soenen, M Baracchi, R De-Corte, L Labey, B Innocenti. "Stemmed TKA in a femur with a total hip arthroplasty: is there a safe distance between the stem tips?". *J Arthroplasty.* 2013,28:1437-45.

[22] D Waanders, Ds Janssen, M A Miller, K A Mann, Ni Verdonschot. “Fatigue creep damage at the cement–bone interface: An experimental and a micro-mechanical finite element study”. *J Biomech.* 2009,42:2513-19.

[23] B Innocenti, O F Bilgen, L Labey, G H van Lenthe, J Vander Sloten, F Catani. Load Sharing and Ligament Strains in Balanced, Overstuffed and Understuffed UKA”. *J Arthroplasty.* 2014,29:1491–8.

[24] F Catani, B Innocenti, C Belvedere, A Ensini, A Leardini. “The Mark Coventry Award: Articular contact estimation in TKA using in vivo kinematics and finite element analysis. *Clin Orthop Relat Res.* 2010,468:19-28.

[25] B Innocenti, L Labey, A Kamali, W Pascale, S Pianigiani. "Development and validation of a wear model to predict polyethylene wear in a total knee arthroplasty: a finite element analysis". *Lubricants.* 2014,2:193-205.

In: New Developments in Knee Prosthesis Research
Editor: Janice Stewart
ISBN: 978-1-63482-700-3

Chapter 5

Patient Specific Instrument in Total Knee Arthroplasty

Daniele Mazza**, Raffaele Iorio, Matteo Guzzini, Edoardo Monaco, Fabio Conteduca and Andrea Ferretti
Orthopaedic Unit and "Kirk Kilgour" Sports Injury Centre,
S. Andrea Hospital, University of Rome "Sapienza", Italy

Abstract

Purpose: In recent years, patient-specific instruments (PSI) has been introduced with the aim to reduce the overall costs of the implants, minimising the size and number of instruments required, and also reducing surgery time. The purpose of this study was to perform a review of the current literature, as well as to report about our personal experience, to assess reliability of patient specific instrument system in total knee arthroplasty (TKA). Method: A literature review was conducted of PSI system reviewing articles related to coronal alignment, clinical knee and function scores, cost, patient satisfaction and complications. Results: Studies have reported incidences of coronal alignment ≥3° from neutral in TKAs performed with patient-specific cutting guides ranging from 6 % to 31 %. Conclusion: PSI seem not to be able to result in the same degree of accuracy as for the CAS system, while comparing well with standard manual technique with respect to component positioning and overall lower axis, in particular in the sagittal plane.

In cases in which custom-made cutting jigs were used, we recommend performing an accurate control of the alignment before and after any cuts and in any further step of the procedure, in order to avoid possible outliers.

* Corresponding author: Daniele Mazza: E-mail: daniele.mazza@hotmail.it.

Introduction

Total knee arthroplasty (TKA) is one of the most successful orthopedic procedures restoring a significant degree of function in arthritic knees in most cases. However, errors in surgical technique and component placement can compromise the long-term performance [1]. It has been proven that one of the most important factors influencing the longevity of implants in TKA is the restoration of mechanical axis, as deviations of greater than 3° of varus/valgus in the mechanical axis lead to poor survivorship because of the accelerated wear as a result of abnormal stresses at the bearing surfaces [2]. The use of computer-assisted surgery (CAS) in TKA results in better coronal alignment of the leg and the implants compared to TKA performed using the standard technique [3]. However, the majority of published studies have not found statistically significant differences between CAS and conventional TKA based on the Knee Society Score (KSS), Western Ontario and McMaster Universities Osteoarthritis Index (WOMAC) or University of California Los Angeles activity score (UCLA). Only one prospective study [4] reported better 5-year KSS results in the CAS TKA group. Moreover, the duration of surgery performed with computer navigation was significantly longer. This is due in part to the surgical technique which requires the placement of the reference arrays, digitization of the knee, and waiting for the computer to work out the algorithms [5]. In recent years, patient-specific instruments (PSI) has been introduced with the aim to reduce the overall costs of the implants, minimising the size and number of instruments required, and also reducing surgery time. PSI uses anatomical data, as detected by pre-operative axial computed tomography (CT) or magnetic resonance imaging (MRI), to create disposable cutting jigs individualized to the patient's unique anatomy. However previous studies [6, 7] documented an only fair accuracy of the method with a consistent risk of error of more than 2°, especially in the sagittal plane.

PSI System

Patient-specific instruments (PSI) were recently introduced as a new technology, to pursue the same goal of navigation in increasing the accuracy of the surgical technique, avoiding the practical issues related to the complexity of the CAS, such as the costs, surgical time and the learning curve related to the procedure. The pre-operative planning of the TKA procedure is outsourced to engineers who identify the anatomical landmarks needed for components alignment on CT/MRI based 3D models, therefore transferring the informations to patient-specific instruments that can be used during surgery. These instruments, created by laser sintering, can be produced in the most complex forms and are thus patient specific [8].

This technology gained widespread acceptance in dental surgery and was gradually introduced in TKA. Using a preoperative CT or MRI scan, disposable cutting blocks are produced. Thienpont et al. [9] showed that the total volume of PSI in Europe for 2012 was 17,515 total knee arthroplasty and 82,556 TKA worldwide. The seven companies which provided PSI are by alphabetical order: Biomet (Warsaw, US), DuPuy-Synthes (Warsaw, US), Medacta (Castel San Pietro, Switzerland), Smith and Nephew (Memphis, US), Stryker (Mahwah, US), Wright Medical (Memphis, US) and Zimmer (Warsaw, US). Biomet was the number one in volume, both in Europe as worldwide with their Signature system. Biomet represented 27 % of the market share in PSI worldwide.

Pre-Operative Data

Bone models generated from CT data have been shown to be more accurate and smooth in their external surface boundaries than MRI-generated models [10]. By contrast, the segmentation process of the images can be performed on the surface of the articular cartilage using MRI data, whereas the articular cartilage surface cannot be estimated using CT data. A study of cadaveric knees demonstrated that the patient-matched cutting block based on CT imaging shows good rotational alignment accuracy except for one specimen with badly damaged cartilage [11]. Because the patient-specific guide based on CT images was created using a bone model without the cartilage, the guide did not make contact the local area of the articular surface where the cartilage was worn away. In varus deformity osteoarthritis, the articular cartilage has already been worn away at the distal part of medial femoral condyle and the proximal part of medial tibial plateau.

Therefore, the residual cartilage evaluation seemed to influence the alignment particularly on the coronal plane. Because the purpose of undergoing MRI was to construct three-dimensional bone models, the patient had to be immobilized from the start to the end of the procedure to avoid motion artifacts. Conversely, there was considerable concern regarding the radiation dose from CT to create the patient-specific guide. Although it is still unknown whether the cancer risk for TKA patients after CT scan exposure increases, and, CT scans should be limited to definite situations in order to avoid unnecessary radiation exposure [12]. If the results obtained using the patient-specific guide based on CT images were the same as those based on MRI, the radiation dose from modern CT scanners might be of little concern for cases that could not receive MRI because of metallic hardware or motion artifacts.

Cost Analysis

DeHaan et al. analyzed costs of PSI [13]. Of the variables assessed for patient-specific TKAs, the two that added cost were the price of the pre-operative advanced imaging ($430–$1360) and the cost of the custom cutting blocks ($500). The other variables measured all served to save money and increase efficiency for the patient-specific instrumentation group: shorter operating room time, fewer instrument trays requiring sterilization, and a shorter operating room turnover time. The 20.4 min shorter operating room time for the patient-specific TKA group provided an average cost savings of $1326 (20.4 min × $65/min) per case when compared to conventional TKA.

Similarly, arthroplasty done with patient-specific instrumentation used 4 fewer instrument trays than with conventional instrumentation, and would thus provide an additional cost savings of $240 (4 trays × $60/tray) per case. Unfortunately, the financial impact of a 42% shorter operating room turnover time could not be quantified; however, this increased efficiency would provide additional cost savings to the hospital through money saved in fewer nursing and surgical staff hours, along with the potential of having additional time for more surgical cases. Thus, they found that the routine use of patient-specific instrumentation in TKA added between $830 and $1860 per case based on the cost of the advanced imaging and the prefabricated cutting blocks. However, shorter operating room time and the use of less surgical trays per case saved $1566 per case, along with the additional variable of increased turnover time efficiency. Thus, routine use of patient-specific instrumentation does not appear to add to the overall cost to primary TKA, but can actually result in significant cost savings dependent upon which imaging center is used.

Blood Loss

Spencer et al. [14] analyzed the results of 30 TKA's performed with the OtisMed custom-fit technique and compared them to a matched cohort operated on using conventional alignment guides. There were no differences in blood loss, and there was a mean decrease in tourniquet time of 14 % compared to a cohort of patients with conventional knee replacements (80 ± 17 vs 93 ± 12 min). Chareancholvanich et al. [15] randomized 80 patients to undergo TKR with PSG or conventional instrumentation and found that the operating time was reduced by a mean 5.1 min ($p = 0.019$), without tangible differences in postoperative blood loss (p = n.s.) or need for blood transfusion (p = n.s.). Noble et al. carried out prospective randomized study comparing Visionnaire (15 patients) to standard instrumentation (14 patients). They found a small although significant reduction in the length of hospital stay (59.2 vs 66.9 h, n.s.) and operative time (121.4 vs 128.1 min, $p < 0.048$). They found no significant difference in blood loss (71 vs 62.5 mL, n.s.). Boonen et al. [16] reported significantly lower blood loss and shorter operation time with the PSG system than with the conventional system. Blood loss being 100 mL less and operation time being 5 min shorter.

Final Alignment

The peer-reviewed literature on PSI is still limited with only a few high-quality studies available. The initial papers by early adopters of the technology were globally showing a mean mechanical axis comparable to conventional surgery with a lower rate of outliers in the coronal plane, but without significant difference [8, 17]. Subsequently, a few retrospective studies about a MRI-based system [6, 7], and a recent randomized controlled trial, where different PSI systems were controlled with navigation during surgery, did not show convincing evidence for three-plane alignment superiority for PSI in comparison with standard technique [8].

Previous studies have reported incidences of coronal alignment ≥3° from neutral in TKAs performed with patient-specific cutting guides ranging from 6 % [18] to 31 % [19] (Table 1). Moreover, the PSI system did not demonstrate a marked improvement in the incidence of outliers in final coronal alignment, comparing poorly with computer-assisted navigation (9 %), with rates of outliers to technique (31.8 %) [20]. Bali et al. [17] shared their initial experience with use of PSI in 32 TKAs. At 6 weeks, long-leg radiographs were obtained to evaluate the coronal alignment and twenty-nine of the 32 knees (90.6%) had a mechanical axis restored to within 3° of neutral.

The authors concluded that custom-fit system in TKA was found to be as accurate in restoring the postoperative alignment as the standard TKA. Noble et al. [21] compared the value of the new mechanically aligned patient-matched instrument system for total knee arthroplasty to that of standard TKA surgical instrumentation. Mechanical alignment was significantly closer to neutral zero in the PSI group (1.7° range 0-6° vs 2.8° range 0-5°).

Table 1. Comparative studies for PSI assessments

Study	Patient	System	Implant	Method	HKA	CTA	CFA	STA	SFA
Nam et al. [22] 2013	41	Signature Biomet (MRI)	Vanguard Complete Knee System (Biomet)	X-Rays	0.8° ± 2.9° 29.3% outliers	0.4° ± 1.6° 12.8% outliers	0.1° ± 1.5° 9.8% outliers	NA	NA
Chen et al. [19] 2013	29	Zimmer PSI system (MRI)	Zimmer Nexgen LPS system	X-Rays	179.2 ± 3.4 9 outliers (31%)	89.8 ± 1.9 3outliers (10%)	89.9 ± 2.1 2 outliers (7%)	84.2 ± 3.4 7 outliers (24%)	87.7 ± 2.6 7 outliers (24%)
Boonen et al. [16] 2013	45	Signature Biomet (MRI)	Vanguard Complete Knee System (Biomet)	X-Rays	179°± 2.8 30% outliers	90°±2.0 9% outliers	89°±2.1 13% outliers	92°±3.2 33% outliers	96°±5 49% outliers
Parratte et al. [32] 2013	20	Zimmer PSI system (MRI)	Zimmer Nexgen LPS system	X-Rays	179° (171–185) 4 outliers (20%)	89.1 (85–96)	90.1 (84–83)	5.9 (3–9)	8.15 (2–14)
Pietsch et al. [18] 2013	50	Zimmer PSI system (MRI)	Zimmer Nexgen LPS system	X-Rays	3 outliers (6%)	4 outliers (8%)	5 outliers (10%)	3 outliers (6%)	3 outliers (6%)
Daniilidis et al. [23] 2013	150	Visionaire PSI Smith and Nephew (MRI)	Genesis II (Smith and Nephew)	X-Rays	178.4 ± 1.5 14 outliers (9.3%)	NA	NA	NA	NA
Vundelinckx et al. [33] 2013	31	Visionaire PSI Smith and Nephew (MRI)	Genesis II (Smith and Nephew)	X-Rays	183±2.59	NA	NA	NA	NA
Koch et al. [25] 2013	301	MyKnee Medacta (CT)	GMK (Medacta)	X-Rays	180.1° ± 2.0 34 outliers (11.7%)	11 outliers (3.8%)	13 outliers (4.5%)	37 outliers (12.3%)	27 outliers (9%)
Scholes et al. [26] 2013	30	Zimmer PSI system (MRI)	Zimmer Nexgen LPS system	Nav	179.5° 8 outliers (27%)	NA	NA	NA	NA

Table 1. (Continued)

Study	Patient	System	Implant	Method	HKA	CTA	CFA	STA	SFA
Lustig et al. [27] 2013	60	Visionaire Smithand Nephew (MRI)	Genesis II (S and N)	Nav	179.8 20.9% ouliers	NA	NA	NA	NA
Daniilidis et al. [34] 2012	124	Visionaire Smith and Nephew (MRI)	Genesis II (Smith and Nephew)	X-Rays	178.5±1.7 11 outliers (11%)	NA	NA	NA	NA
Bali et al. [17] 2012	32	Visionaire Smith and Nephew (MRI)	Genesis II (Smith and Nephew)	X-Rays	179.9 3 outliers (9.4%)	NA	NA	NA	NA
Ng et al. [24] 2012	569	Signature Biomet (MRI)	Vanguard Complete Knee System (Biomet)	X-Rays	180.6° 9% outliers	89.9° 10% outliers	90.7° 22% outliers	NA	NA
Conteduca et al. [7] 2012	12	Visionaire Smith and Nephew (MRI)	Journey BCS (S and N)	Nav	NA	1.2°±1.5 2 outliers (16%)	1.2°±0.6 2 outliers (16%)	3.8°±2.4 9 outliers (75%)	+0.5°±2.15 3 outliers (25%)
Noble et al. [21] 2012	15	Visionaire Smith and Nephew (MRI)	Legion Total Knee System (Smith and Nephew)	X-Rays	181.7	NA	NA	NA	NA
Nunley et al. [35] 2012	57	Vanguard total knee system (Biomet) (MRI)	Signature system (Biomet)	CT-scan	26% outliers	NA	NA	NA	NA

HKA=hip-knee-ankle angle.
CTA=coronal tibial angle.
CFA=coronal femoral angle.
STA=sagittal tibial angle.
SFA=sagittal femoral angle.

The results of the this randomized study support the value of patient-matched cutting blocks. However this study is only representative of 1 surgeon's experience. Nam et al. [22] compared the alignment accuracy of PSI to an imageless CAS system in TKA. In the PSI cohort, 70.7% of patients had an overall alignment within 3° of a neutral mechanical axis (vs. 92.7% with CAS), 87.8% had a tibial component alignment within 2° of perpendicular to the tibial mechanical axis (vs. 100% with CAS), and 90.2% had a femoral component alignment within 2° of perpendicular to the femoral mechanical axis (vs. 100% with CAS).

The author concluded that, while PSI techniques appear sound in principle, this system did not obtain the same degree of overall mechanical and tibial component alignment accuracy as a CAS technique.

Daniilidis et al. [23] determined whether PSI would lead to a hip-knee-ankle (HKA) angle within ±3° of the ideal alignment of 180°. The average HKA changed from 173.7°±3.9 preoperatively to 178.4±1.5° postoperatively. The rate of ±3° and ±5° HKA outliers was 11 % and 3 %, respectively. On the basis of their data, authors showed that these results also reconfirm the conclusion that this specific technology is effective in addressing the issue of malalignment.

Ng et al. [24] compared the effectiveness of MRI-based patient-specific positioning guides to manual instrumentation with intra-medullary femoral and extra-medullary tibial guides in restoring the mechanical axis of the extremity and achieving neutral coronal alignment of the femoral and tibial components. The overall mean HKA angle for patient-specific positioning guides (180.6°) was similar to manual instrumentation (181.1°), but there were a statistically fewer ± 3° HKA angle outliers with patient-specific positioning guides (9%) than with manual instrumentation (22%).

By our knowledge only one study analyzed CT-based system. Koch et al. [25] showed that the postoperative average HKA angle of a CT-based system was 180.1° ± 2.0°.

In the frontal plane a total of 12.4 % of outliers >3°, for the tibial components 4.1 % of outliers >3° and for the femoral components 4.8 % of outliers >3° were measured. Comparing the outcome of this study with the data from the literature [20], there does not seem to be any difference compared to computer-assisted surgery.

Based on these studies we could speculate that the MRI-based PSI system was not able to obtain the same degree of accuracy as the CAS system, with respect to both the tibial component and overall lower extremity axis in particular in sagittal plane. While themean valuesare comparable to most reports of TKAs performed using conventional intramedullary and extra-medullary alignment methods, it falls far below the accuracy reported with CAS techniques [20]. However in most cases the authors failed to report about recut performed during surgery to correct possible misalignment related to inaccuracy of the guided cut.

Moreover these studies only evaluated the alignment in the coronal plane, not considering possible malposition in the sagittal plane that may play a significant role in the maximal post-operative flexion and in the polyethylene wears. Another limitation of previous studies is that the accuracy of the PSI was evaluated using post-operative x-rays, whose data can be influenced by several factor other than accuracy of the cutting guide (sawing errors, cut adjustment, final impaction technique). Computer navigation provides the only real-time method for assessing alignment of system and to our knowledge only few studies [6, 7, 26, 27, 28] used this to evaluate the PSI.

Lustig et al. [27] used intra-operative computer navigation to evaluate the accuracy of the cutting blocks in the coronal and sagittal planes. The PSI would have placed 79.3% of the sample within ±3° of the preoperative plan in the coronal plane, while the sagittal alignment results within ±3 were 54.5%.

Their results are very similar to the data previously reported by us [6, 7]. Even more disappointing were the results of Klatt et al. [28] who used an image-free computer navigation system to evaluate the alignment of the components that was more than 3° off of mechanical axis in all cases.

On the basis of their data, author showed that the custom cutting jigs have the potential to place the components outside of the accepted range of alignment and even place the components out of the accepted alignment range.

In a similar study Scholes et al. [26] assessed reliability of PSI in TKA using imageless computer navigation. The error between in-theatre measurements and pre-operative plan for the femoral and tibial components exceeded 3° for 3% and 17 % of the sample respectively, while the error for total coronal alignment exceeded 3° for 27 % of the sample.

The authors concluded that alignment with PSI patient-specific cutting guides, assessed by computer navigation, is not accurate. To prevent unnecessary increases in the incidence of malalignment in TKA, it is recommended that these devices should not be used without verification of alignment.

Our Experience

We started using PSI in 2011 after a consistent experience with navigation in TKA [6, 7; 29-31]. In a recent study [7] we evaluated the accuracy of a patient-specific instrumentation as assessed by the intra-operative use of knee navigation software during the surgical procedure.

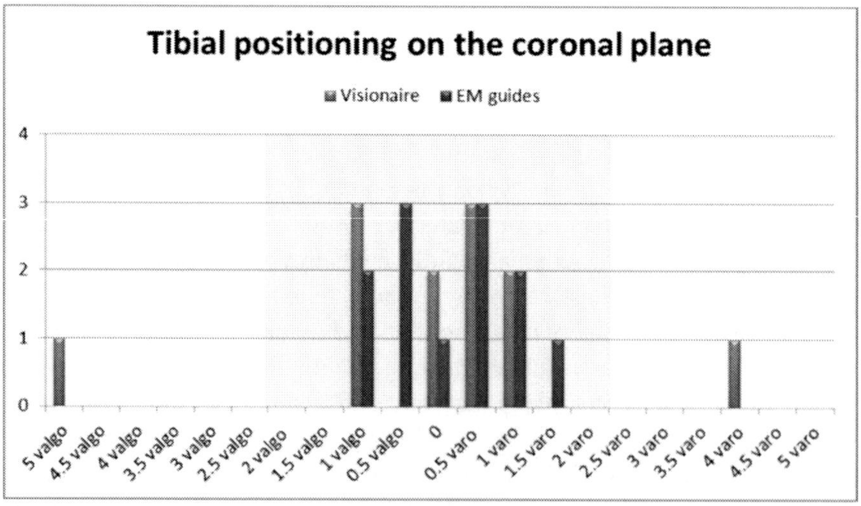

Figure 1. (A) EM guide vs VISIONAIRE on the coronal plane.

Ten satisfactory alignments (83.3%) were obtained on the tibial coronal plane. A correct alignment was achieved on the tibial sagittal plane in 5 patients only (41.6%). On the femur, a correct alignment was obtained for 11 measurements (92.6 %) in the coronal plane and in 9

(71 %) in the sagittal plane. We also evaluate the accuracy of VISIONAIRE (Smith and Nephew Inc., Memphis, TN, US) in comparison with extra-medullary (EM) tibial instrumentation by analyzing data as detected by intra-operative use of knee navigation software. In the coronal plane the mean deviation of the EM tibial guides from the ideal alignment (0°) was 0.7°±0.39 and of the VISIONAIRE was 1.2°±1.5 (P=0.22). In the sagittal plane the mean deviation of the EM tibial guides from 3° of posterior slope was -1.6°±1.7° and of the VISIONAIRE was +1.1°±4.2 (P<0.05). Negative values indicate a more posterior slope from the ideal and positive values an anterior slope [6]. All data were showed in figure 1A, 1B, 2A, 2B.

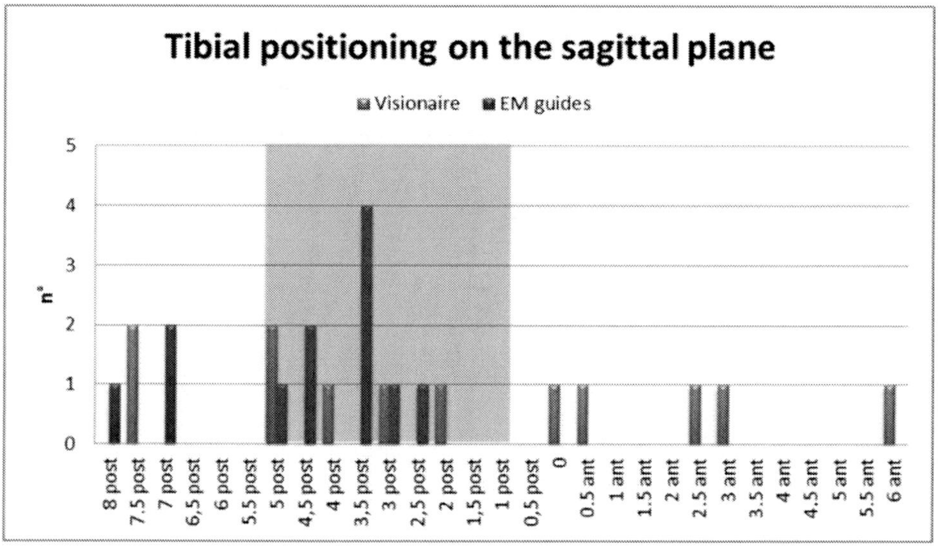

Figure 1. (B) EM guide vs VISIONAIRE on the sagittal plane.

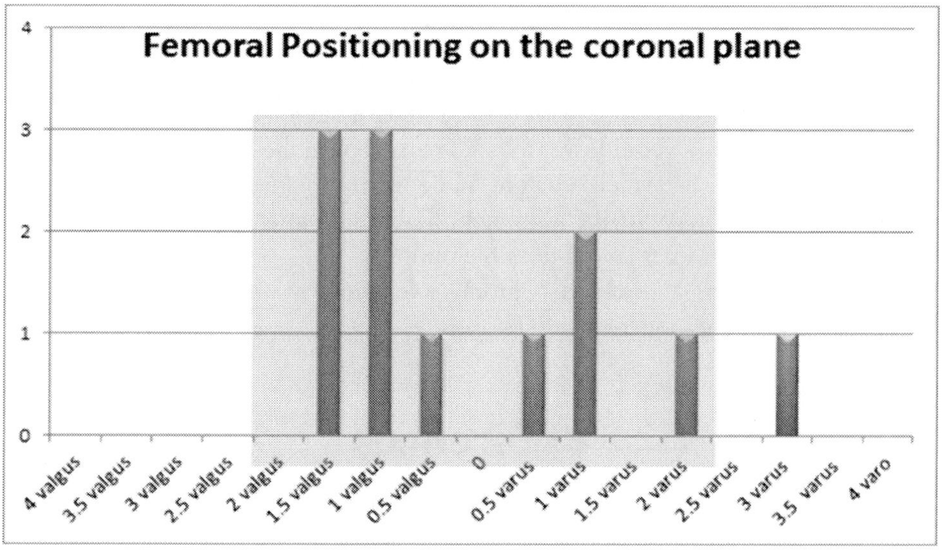

Figure 2. (A) The alignment on the coronal femoral plane.

These studies documented only a fair accuracy of the method with a consistent risk of error of more of 3° especially in the sagittal plane. We could speculate that the problem in the sagittal plane was due to the fact that the pre-operative protocol does not include a lateral X-ray projection of the knee and only includes an AP standing X-ray of the straight leg and MRI.

Conclusion

Patient specific instruments have been introduced to reduce the surgical time, the overall costs of the implants, minimising the size and number of instruments required.

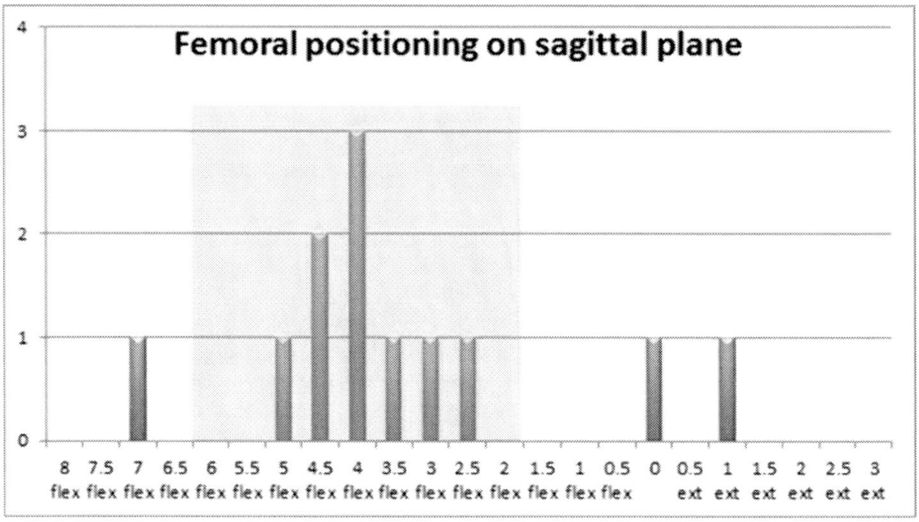

Figure 2. (B) The alignment on the sagittal femoral plane.

However current PSI seem not to be able to result in the same degree of accuracy as for the CAS system, while comparing well with standard manual technique with respect to component positioning and overall lower axis, in particular in the sagittal plane.

Nowadays, in cases in which custom-made cutting jigswere used, we recommend performing an accurate control of the alignment before and after any cuts and in any further step of the procedure, in order to avoid possible outliers.

Therefore even if PSI appears as a promise technology, their accuracy could be still improved, possibly leading to greater reliability.

References

[1] Jeffery, R. S., Morris, R. W., Denham, R. A. (1991) Coronal alignment after total knee replacement. *J. Bone Joint Surg. Br.* Sep;73(5):709-714.

[2] Perillo-Marcone, A., Barrett, D. S., Taylor, M. (2000) The importance of tibial alignment: finite element analysis of tibial malalignment. *J. Arthroplasty.* Dec;15(8): 1020-1027.

[3] Lützner, J., Dexel, J., Kirschner, S. (2013) No difference between computer-assisted and conventional total knee arthroplasty: five-year results of a prospective randomized study. *Knee Surg. Sports Traumatol. Arthrosc.* Oct;21(10):2241-2247.

[4] Hoffart, H. E., Langenstein, E., Vasak, N. (2012) A prospective study comparing the functional outcome of computer-assisted and conventional total knee replacement. *J. Bone Joint Surg. Br.* Feb;94(2): 194-199.

[5] Chin, P. L., Yang, K. Y., Yeo, S. J., Lo, N. N. (2005) Randomized control trial comparing radiographic total knee arthroplasty implant placement using computer navigation versus conventional technique. *J. Arthroplasty.* Aug;20(5):618-626.

[6] Conteduca, F., Iorio, R., Mazza, D., Caperna, L., Bolle, G., Argento, G., Ferretti, A. (2012) Are MRI-based, patient matched cutting jigs as accurate as the tibial guides? *Int. Orthop.* Aug;36(8):1589-1593.

[7] Conteduca, F., Iorio, R., Mazza, D., Caperna, L., Bolle, G., Argento, G., Ferretti, A. (2013) Evaluation of the accuracy of a patient-specific instrumentation by navigation. *Knee Surg. Sports Traumatol. Arthrosc.* Oct;21(10):2194-2199.

[8] Victor, J., Dujardin, J., Vandenneucker, H., Arnout, N., Bellemans, J. (2013) Patient-specific Guides Do Not Improve Accuracy in Total Knee Arthroplasty: A Prospective Randomized Controlled Trial. *Clin. Orthop. Relat. Res.* Apr. 25. PubMed PMID: 23616267.

[9] Thienpont, E., Bellemans, J., Delport, H., Van Overschelde, P., Stuyts, B., Brabants, K., Victor, J. (2013) Patient-specific instruments: industry's innovation with a surgeon's interest. *Knee Surg. Sports Traumatol. Arthrosc.* Oct;21(10):2227-2233.

[10] White, D., Chelule, K. L., Seedhom, B. B. (2008) Accuracy of MRI vs CT imaging with particular reference to patient specific templates for total knee replacement surgery. *Int. J. Med. Robot* Sep;4(3):224–31.

[11] Tibesku, C. O., Innocenti, B., Wong, P., Salehi, A., Labey, L. (2012) Can CT-based patient-matched instrumentation achieve consistent rotational alignment in knee arthroplasty? *Arch. Orthop. Trauma Surg.* Feb;132(2):171–7.

[12] Eisenberg, M. J., Afilalo, J., Lawler, P. R., Abrahamowicz, M., Richard, H., Pilote, L. (2011) Cancer risk related to low-dose ionizing radiation from cardiac imaging in patients after acute myocardial infarction. *CMAJ* Mar. 8 2011;183(4):430–6.

[13] DeHaan, A. M., Adams, J. R., DeHart, M. L., Huff, T. W. (2014) Patient-specific versus conventional instrumentation for total knee arthroplasty: peri-operative and cost differences. *J. Arthroplasty.* Nov;29(11):2065-9.

[14] Spencer, B. A., Mont, M. A., McGrath, M. S., et al. (2009) Initial experience with custom-fit total knee replacement: intra-operative events and long-leg coronal alignment. *Int. Orthop.*; 33(6):1571.

[15] Chareancholvanich, K., Narkbunnam, R., Pornrattanameneegwong, C. (2013) A prospective andomised controlled study of patient-specific cutting guides compared with conventional instrumentation in total knee replacement. *J. Bone Joint Surg.* Br; 95B(3):354.

[16] Boonen, B., Schotanus, M. G. M., Kerens, B., et al. (2013) Intra-operative results and radiological outcome of conventional and patient-specific surgery in total knee

arthroplasty: amulticentre, randomized controlled trial. *Knee Surg. Sports Traumatol. Arthrosc.*; 21(10):2206.

[17] Bali, K., Walker, P., Bruce, W. (2012) Custom-fit total knee arthroplasty: our initial experience in 32 knees. *J. Arthroplasty*. Jun; 27(6):1149-1154.

[18] Pietsch, M., Djahani, O., Hochegger, M., Plattner, F., Hofmann, S. (2013) Patient-specific total knee arthroplasty: the importance of planning by the surgeon. *Knee Surg. Sports Traumatol. Arthrosc*. Oct; 21(10):2220-2226.

[19] Chen, J. Y., Yeo, S. J., Yew, A. K., Tay, D. K., Chia, S. L., Lo, N. N., Chin, P. L. (2013) The radiological outcomes of patient-specific instrumentation versus conventional total knee arthroplasty. *Knee Surg. Sports Traumatol. Arthrosc.* Aug. 31. PubMed PMID: 23996069.

[20] Mason, J. B., Fehring, T. K., Estok, R., Banel, D., Fahrbach, K. (2007) Meta-analysis of alignment outcomes in computer-assisted total knee arthroplasty surgery. *J. Arthroplasty*. Dec;22(8):1097-1106.

[21] Noble, J. W. Jr, Moore, C. A., Liu, N. (2012) The value of patient-matched instrumentation in total knee arthroplasty. *J. Arthroplasty*. Jan; 27(1):153-155.

[22] Nam, D., Maher, P. A., Rebolledo, B. J., Nawabi, D. H., McLawhorn, A. S., Pearle, A. D. (2013) Patient specific cutting guides versus an imageless, computer-assisted surgery system in total knee arthroplasty. *Knee*. Aug; 20(4):263-267.

[23] Daniilidis, K., Tibesku, C. O. (2013) A comparison of conventional and patient-specific instruments in total knee arthroplasty. *Int. Orthop.* Jul. 31. PubMed PMID: 23900384.

[24] Ng, V. Y., DeClaire, J. H., Berend, K. R., Gulick, B. C., Lombardi, A. V. Jr (2012) Improved accuracy of alignment with patient-specific positioning guides compared with manual instrumentation in TKA. *Clin. Orthop. Relat. Res*. Jan;470(1):99-107.

[25] Koch, P. P., Müller, D., Pisan, M., Fucentese, S. F. (2013) Radiographic accuracy in TKA with a CT-based patient-specific cutting block technique. *Knee Surg. Sports Traumatol. Arthrosc*. Oct;21(10):2200-5.

[26] Scholes, C., Sahni, V., Lustig, S., Parker, D. A., Coolican, M. R. (2013) Patient-specific instrumentation for total knee arthroplasty does not match the pre-operative plan as assessed by intra-operative computer-assisted navigation. *Knee Surg. Sports Traumatol. Arthrosc*. Sep. 17. PubMed PMID: 24042965.

[27] Lustig, S., Scholes, C. J., Oussedik, S., Kinzel, V., Coolican, M. R., Parker, D. A. (2013) Unsatisfactory Accuracy with VISIONAIRE Patient-Specific Cutting Jigs for Total Knee Arthroplasty. *J. Arthroplasty.* Jul. 25. PubMed PMID: 23891059.

[28] Klatt, B. A., Goyal, N., Austin, M. S., Hozack, W. J. (2008) Custom-fit total knee arthroplasty (Otis Knee) results in malalignment. *J. Arthroplasty.* Jan;23(1):26-29.

[29] Conteduca, F., Massai, F., Iorio, R., Zanzotto, E., Luzon, D., Ferretti, A. (2009) Blood loss in computer-assisted mobile bearing total knee arthroplasty. A comparison of computer-assisted surgery with a conventional technique. *Int. Orthop*. Dec;33(6):1609-1613.

[30] Iorio, R., Bolle, G., Conteduca, F., Valeo, L., Conteduca, J., Mazza, D., Ferretti, A. (2013) Accuracy of manual instrumentation of tibial cutting guide in total knee arthroplasty. *Knee Surg. Sports Traumatol. Arthrosc*. Oct;21(10):2296-2300.

[31] Iorio, R., Mazza, D., Bolle, G., Conteduca, J., Redler, A., Conteduca, F., Ferretti, A. (2013) Computer-assisted surgery: a teacher of TKAs. *Knee*. Aug;20(4):232-235.

[32] Parratte, S., Blanc, G., Boussemart, T., Ollivier, M., Le Corroller, T., Argenson, J. N. (2013) Rotation in total knee arthroplasty: no difference between patient-specific and conventional instrumentation. *Knee Surg. Sports Traumatol. Arthrosc.* Oct;21(10): 2213-2219.

[33] Vundelinckx, B. J., Bruckers, L., De Mulder, K., De Schepper, J., Van Esbroeck, G. (2013) Functional and radiographic short-term outcome evaluation of the Visionaire system, a patient-matched instrumentation system for total knee arthroplasty. *J. Arthroplasty*. 2013 Jun;28(6):964-970.

[34] Daniilidis, K., Tibesku, C. O. (2013) Frontal plane alignment after total knee arthroplasty using patient-specific instruments. *Int. Orthop*. Jan;37(1):45-50.

[35] Nunley, R. M., Ellison, B. S., Ruh, E. L., Williams, B. M., Foreman, K., Ford, A. D., Barrack, R. L. (2012) Are patient-specific cutting blocks cost-effective for total knee arthroplasty? *Clin. Orthop. Relat. Res*. Mar; 470(3):889-94.

In: New Developments in Knee Prosthesis Research
Editor: Janice Stewart
ISBN: 978-1-63482-700-3

Chapter 6

Screening and Decolonization of MRSA Among Knee Joint Arthroplasty Patients: Efficacy, Cost-Effectiveness and Durability

E. Carlos Rodriguez-Merchan[*]
Professor, Department of Orthopedic Surgery
La Paz University Hospital, Madrid, Spain

Abstract

Background: Although some have advocated screening (nasal swab using polymerase chain reaction (PCR)-based testing), followed by decolonization using a 5 to 14-days course of nasal mucopirocin (2 per cent nasal ointment) for methicillin resistant *Staphylococcus aureus* (MRSA), it is unclear whether screening and decolonization (S&D) among knee joint arthroplasty patients reduce surgical site infections (SSIs)

Purpose: The purpose of this chapter is to review the literature with the aim of answering the following three questions: 1) Is S&D effective in reducing the rate of postoperative infection after elective knee joint arthroplasty? 2) Is S&D cost-effective? 3) What is the durability of decolonization?

Methods: The search engines were MedLine (PubMed), Google Scholar and the Cochrane Library. The keywords used were: preoperative MRSA screening. 8008 papers were found until 25 October 2014 (7910 in Google Scholar, 97 in MedLine and one in the Cochrane Library). Of those, only eighteen were selected and reviewed because they were strictly focused on the question of this article.

Results: The types of studies reported have a low level of evidence (level III, level IV). Most of them are prospective case series (level IV), although some of them are systematic reviews of level III studies. Regarding the efficacy of decolonization, the literature shows a tendency toward fewer MRSA infections after elective knee joint

[*] e-mail address: ecrmerchan@gmx.es

arthroplasty. Decolonization has shown to be strongly cost-effective. Regarding the durability of decolonization, in a study 33% of postoperative arthroplasty patients tested positive for SA colonization at 3 to 30 months after surgery.

Conclusions: The review of the literature found a tendency toward fewer MRSA infections after knee joint arthroplasty when S&D was used. Decolonization is strongly cost-effective procedure. Regarding the durability of decolonization, 33% of patients tested positive for MRSA 3 to 30 months after surgery. However, most of these studies were underpowered. Larger, randomized, controlled studies are needed to confirm the apparent efficacy of decolonization.

Keywords: knee, joint arthroplasty, *Staphylococcus aureus*, postoperative infection, screening and decolonization, efficacy, cost-effectiveness, durability

Introduction

Staphylococcus aureus (SA) is the most common organism responsible for orthopaedic surgical site infections (SSIs) after elective joint arthroplasty. Patients who are carriers for methicillin resistant *Staphylococcus aureus* (MRSA) have a higher likelihood of having invasive MRSA infections [1].

Some have suggested that screening and decolonization (S&D) of all patients having elective joint arthroplasty will decrease the incidence of postoperative infections [2]. They believe that a prescreening program (nasal swab using polymerase chain reaction (PCR)-based testing), followed by an appropriate eradication using a 5 to 14-days course of nasal mucopirocin (2 per cent nasal ointment) will lower the rate of SSIs [3].

Although some authors have advocated S&D [3] [4], it is unclear whether these efforts reduce SSIs [1]. In other words, while some institutions and surgeons have implemented universal S&D on their patients undergoing elective arthroplasty, others remain unconvinced about the efficacy of this process [5].

The purpose of this chapter is to revise the literature with the aim of answering the following three questions: 1) Is S&D of MRSA effective in reducing the incidence of postoperative infection after elective knee joint arthroplasty? 2) Is decolonization cost-effective? 3) What is the durability of decolonization?

Methods

A review has been performed on the role of S&D of MRSA in reducing the incidence of postoperative infection after elective knee joint arthroplasty. The keywords used were: preoperative MRSA screening. The search engines were MedLine (PubMed), Google Scholar and the Cochrane Library. 8008 were found until 25 October 2014 (7910 in Google Scholar, 97 in MedLine and one in the Cochrane Library). Of those, only eighteen were selected and reviewed because they were strictly focused on the question of this article.

Results

The types of studies reported have a low level of evidence (level III, level IV). Most of them are prospective case series (level IV), although some of them are systematic reviews of level III studies. A survey reported by Diekema et al. [6] showed that only sixty percent of physicians reported preoperative screening for *Staphylococcus aureus*. The incidence of nasal carries of MRSA reported in the orthopaedic literature is very variable, ranging from 1.1% to 25% (TABLE 1) [3] [7-14]. Regarding the efficacy of decolonization, the orthopaedic literature has shown a tendency toward fewer MRSA infections after total joint arthroplasty (TABLE 1). In the study of Mehta et al. [15] before implementation of S&D there was a prevalence density rate (MRSA-positive cultures) of 1.23 per 1000 patient-days. After S&D, the rate was 0.83 per 1000 patient-days. Two reports have shown that preoperative S&D of MRSA is strongly cost-effective (incremental cost-effectiveness ratio less than $6,000 per quality-adjusted life year) from the third-party payer perspective even when MRSA prevalence was as low as 1%, decolonization success was as low as 25%, and decolonization costs were as high as $300 per patient [16]. In most scenarios this strategy was economically dominant (ie, less costly and more effective than no screening).

Table 1. Incidence of nasal carriers of MRSA (methicillin-resistant *Staphylococcus aureus*) and reduction of the rate of surgical site infection (SSI) in elective joint arthroplasty. NA=Nonavailable

AUTHOR	INCIDENCE OF NASAL CARRIES OF MRSA (%)	REDUCTION OF THE RATE OF SURGICAL SITE INFECTION (SSI)
Price [7]	6	NA
Pofahl [8]	0.23	From 0.30% to 0%
Bajolet [9]	1.1	NA
Hadley [10]	1.45	From 1.45% to 1.28%
Kim [11]	4.4	From 0.97% to 0.14%
Gupta [12]	6.6	NA
Kelly [13]	0.49	From 0.49% to 0.24%
Savage [3]	18-25	NA
Chen [14]	4.6	From 4.6% to 0%

Routine preoperative S&D of patients undergoing elective joint arthroplasty may under many circumstances save hospitals and third-party payers money while providing health benefits. Slover et al. [17] conducted a Markov decision analysis to assess the cost savings associated with a preoperative MRSA S&D program on hip and knee arthroplasties. They concluded that universal MRSA S&D for hip and knee arthroplasty patients needs to result in only a modest reduction in the SSI rate to be cost saving.

Concerning the durability of decolonization, arthroplasty surgeons must be aware that a decolonization treatment does not guarantee that a patient will remain decolonized in the future [18]. In a study, 33% of postoperative arthroplasty patients tested positive for MRSA colonization at 3 to 30 months after surgery despite preoperative decolonization [18].

Discussion

The purpose of this article was to review the literature with the aim of answering the following the following three questions: 1) Is S&D of MRSA effective in reducing the rate of postoperative infection after elective knee joint arthroplasty? 2) Is decolonization cost-effective? 3) What is the durability of decolonization? The quality of studies reported so far on the topic is poor (low level of evidence, level III, level IV). Most of them are prospective case series (level IV), although some are systematic reviews of level III studies [1-19]. In a survey only sixty percent of physicians reported preoperative screening for *Staphylococcus aureus* [6]. The incidence of nasal carries of MRSA in the orthopaedic literature is very variable, ranging from 1.1% to 25% [4, 7-14]. Regarding the efficacy of decolonization, a reduction of the incidence of postoperative SSI after elective joint arthroplasty has been found in the literature (TABLE 1). The prevalence density rate (MRSA-positive cultures) of 1.23 per 1000 patient-days before decolonization dropped to 0.83 per 1000 patient-days after decolonization [14]. Preoperative MRSA S&D is strongly cost-effective (incremental cost-effectiveness ratio less than $6,000 per quality-adjusted life year) from the third-party payer perspective even when MRSA prevalence was as low as 1%, decolonization success was as low as 25%, and decolonization costs were as high as $300 per patient [16]. A Markov decision analysis showed that universal SA S&D for hip and knee arthroplasty patients needs to result in only a modest reduction in the SSI rate to be cost saving. Concerning the durability of decolonization, arthroplasty surgeons must be aware that a decolonization treatment does not guarantee that a patient will remain decolonized in the future [18]. In a study, 33% of postoperative arthroplasty patients tested positive for MRSA colonization at 3 to 30 months after surgery despite preoperative decolonization [18].

In conclusion, the review of the literature found a tendency toward fewer MRSA SSIs after knee joint arthroplasty when a S&D program was used. However, most of these studies were underpowered. Larger, randomized, controlled studies are needed to confirm the apparent efficacy of decolonization. S&D is a cost-effective procedure. Regarding the durability of decolonization, one third of patients tested positive for SA 3 to 30 months after surgery.

References

[1] Chen AF, Wessel CB, Rao N. Staphylococcus aureus screening and decolonization in orthopaedic surgery and reduction of surgical site infections. *Clin. Orthop. Relat. Res.* 2013;471(7):2383-99.

[2] Shams WE, Rapp RP. Methicillin-resistant staphylococcal infections: an important consideration for orthopedic surgeons. *Orthopedics*. 2004;27(6):565-8.

[3] Savage JW, Anderson PA. An update on modifiable factors to reduce the risk of surgical site infections. *Spine J*. 2013;13(9):1017-29.

[4] Glassner PJ, Slover JD, Bosco JA 3rd, Zuckerman JD. Blood, bugs, and motion - what do we really know in regard to total joint arthroplasty? *Bull NYU Hosp. Jt Dis*. 2011;69(1):73-80.

[5] Parvizi J. CORR insights: Staphylococcus aureus colonization among arthroplasty patients previously treated by a decolonization protocol: A pilot study. *Clin. Orthop. Relat. Res*. 2013;471:3133-3134.

[6] Diekema D, Johannsson B, Herwaldt L, Beekmann S, Jernigan J, Kallen A, Berrios-Torres S, Polgreen P. Current practice in Staphylococcus aureus screening and decolonization. *Infect. Control Hosp. Epidemiol*. 2011;32(10):1042-4.

[7] Price CS, Williams A, Philips G, Dayton M, Smith W, Morgan S. Staphylococcus aureus nasal colonization in preoperative orthopaedic outpatients. *Clin. Orthop. Relat. Res*. 2008;466(11):2842-7.

[8] Pofahl WE, Goettler CE, Ramsey KM, Cochran MK, Nobles DL, Rotondo MF. Active surveillance screening of MRSA and eradication of the carrier state decreases surgical-site infections caused by MRSA. *J. Am. Coll. Surg*. 2009;208(5):981-6.

[9] Bajolet O, Toussaint E, Diallo S, Vernet-Garnier V, Dehoux E. [Is it possible to detect Staphylococcus aureus colonization or bacteriuria before orthopedic surgery hospitalization?].[Article in French] *Pathol. Biol.* (Paris). 2010;58(2):127-30.

[10] Hadley S, Immerman I, Hutzler L, Slover J, Bosco J. Staphylococcus aureus Decolonization Protocol Decreases Surgical Site Infections for Total Joint Replacement. *Arthritis*. 2010;2010:924518.

[11] Kim DH, Spencer M, Davidson SM, Li L, Shaw JD, Gulczynski D, Hunter DJ, Martha JF, Miley GB, Parazin SJ, Dejoie P, Richmond JC. Institutional prescreening for detection and eradication of methicillin-resistant Staphylococcus aureus in patients undergoing elective orthopaedic surgery. *J. Bone Joint Surg. Am*. 2010;92(9):1820-6.

[12] Gupta K, Strymish J, Abi-Haidar Y, Williams SA, Itani KM. Preoperative nasal methicillin-resistant Staphylococcus aureus status, surgical prophylaxis, and risk-adjusted postoperative outcomes in veterans. *Infect. Control Hosp. Epidemiol*. 2011;32(8):791-6.

[13] Kelly JC, O'Briain DE, Walls R, Lee SI, O'Rourke A, Mc Cabe JP. The role of pre-operative assessment and ringfencing of services in the control of methicillin resistant Staphlococcus aureus infection in orthopaedic patients. *Surgeon*. 2012;10(2):75-9.

[14] Chen AF, Heyl AE, Xu PZ, Rao N, Klatt BA. Preoperative Decolonization Effective at Reducing Staphylococcal Colonization in Total Joint Arthroplasty Patients. *J. Arthroplasty*. 2013 Jul 17. pii: S0883-5403(13)00481-6. doi: 10.1016/j.arth.2013.03.036. [Epub ahead of print]

[15] Mehta S, Hadley S, Hutzler L, Slover J, Phillips M, Bosco JA 3rd. Impact of preoperative MRSA screening and decolonization on hospital-acquired MRSA burden. *Clin. Orthop. Relat. Res*. 2013;471(7):2367-71.

[16] Lee BY, Wiringa AE, Bailey RR, Goyal V, Tsui B, Lewis GJ, Muder RR, Harrison LH. The economic effect of screening orthopedic surgery patients preoperatively for methicillin-resistant Staphylococcus aureus. *Infect. Control Hosp. Epidemiol*. 2010;31(11):1130-8.

[17] Slover J, Haas JP, Quirno M, Phillips MS, Bosco JA 3rd. Cost-effectiveness of a Staphylococcus aureus screening and decolonization program for high-risk orthopedic patients. *J. Arthroplasty*. 2011;26(3):360-5.

[18] Economedes DM, Deirmengian GK, Deirmengian CA. Staphylococcus aureus colonization among arthroplasty patients previously treated by a decolonization protocol: A pilot study. *Clin. Orthop. Relar. Res*. 2013;471:3128-3132.

Index

A

B

C

H

I

J

K

L

M

S

T

U

V

W

X